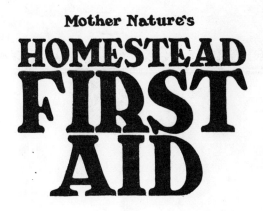

Mother Nature's

HOMESTEAD
FIRST
AID

MOTHER NATURE'S SERIES NUMBER FOUR

Mother Nature's

HOMESTEAD
FIRST
AID

DR. JUDY WILSON

OLIVER PRESS
WILLITS, CALIFORNIA

c1975 152p. il.

Library of Congress Card Number 75-7448

ISBN   0-914400-09-6

Drawings by Nancy Pettitt

Cover by Bruce McCloskey

First Printing May 1975

OLIVER PRESS

1400 Ryan Creek Road

Willits, California 95490

Distributed by

CHARLES SCRIBNER'S SONS

New York

CONTENTS

I   INTRODUCTION vii

II   HOMESTEAD FIRST AID 1

III RESCUSCITATION 19

IV   MUSHROOMS ETC. 33

V   CHEMICAL POISONING 39

VI   BURNS 50

VII CHILDHOOD ACCIDENTS AND ILLNESSES . . 55

VIII EMERGENCY CHILDBIRTHS 63

IX   SNAKE BITE 85

X   SHOCK 99

XI   POISON OAK, IVY, SUMAC 104

XII STRAINS AND SPRAINS 107

XIII BROKEN BONES 113

XIV TRANSPORTATIONS 127

INTRODUCTION

Homesteading is a much used term these days. People are leaving the hectic life of the cities for the quiet and solitude of the country. But even with the advanced knowledge of this day and age, people who live in the country face many of the same problems their grandparents and the early settlers faced.

One of the most critical situations facing the homesteader is that of what to do in case of accident or injury. Not only are people living on farms and mountains far away from hospitals, but the life style is one that lends itself to a large number of potential dangers.

This book is intended to give emergency treatments and perhaps save the lives of the victims of these homestead hazards. It is by no means a medical text, nor can it replace qualified professional treatment. However, use of these procedures can save valuable time and give the victim a chance to get to a hospital or doctor.

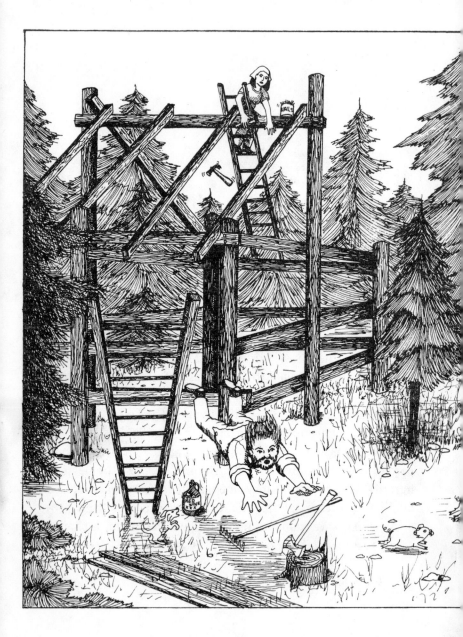

HOMESTEAD FIRST-AID

Homesteads are generally located in areas with poor medical facilities and access to them is over pretty bad roads which are sometimes impassible in the winter. Homesteading also poses more danger of accident than any other lifestyle tolerated in our society. Who besides novice country folk trying to live in the mountains would climb on a homemade ladder, try to hang a twenty foot long log for a ceiling joist on the cabin, or pull the pan on a Chevy pickup to fix a blown rod while the truck is held up by two chunks of firewood?

This book is in no way intended to replace qualified medical help. It is an effort to give the homesteader an accurate and reliable emergency first aid guide in order to help save lives and ease pain. These are emergency procedures only. Most are just good plain horse sense.

Thinking safety, the old cliche, is still the best way of keeping it together. If you fall from a ladder and break some bones you didn't even know you had, not only will it hurt and cost bread you could use on the water system, but chances are your old lady won't be able to get the roof on the cabin before winter by herself.

1

In any emergency it is necessary to stay cool and get into action:

1. If there is bleeding, STOP THE BLEEDING.
2. If there is no breathing, give MOUTH TO MOUTH BREATHING.
3. TREAT FOR SHOCK, in any accident.
4. If the victim is vomiting, MAKE IT POSSIBLE TO DISCHARGE THE VOMIT. A person can drown in his own vomit.

If possible, get immediate help. If you can't, bring the victim to help.

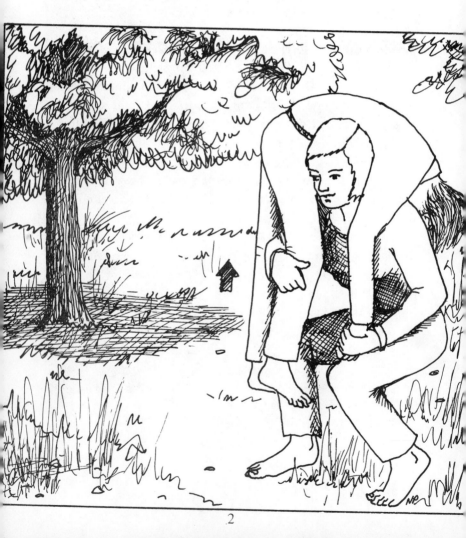

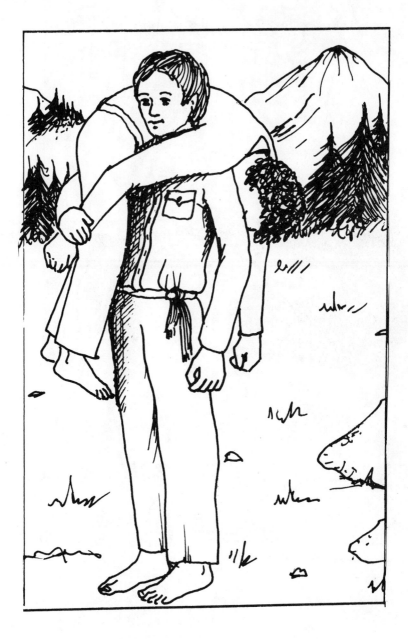

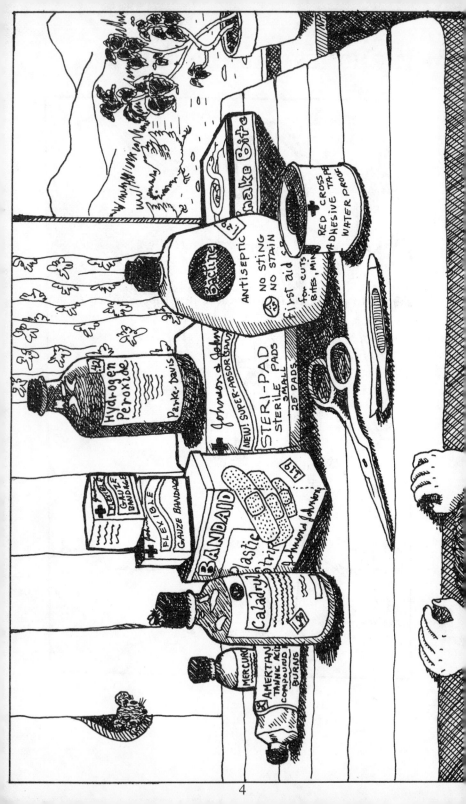

4

THE HOMESTEAD FIRST-AID KIT

There are so many things that the *Whole Earth Catalog* has that you need to put the homestead together that it is easy to forget the first-aid kit, but it should be at the top of the list. If you don't have yours together, get it now, because tomorrow it might be too late.

If you are really remote, or want a more specialized kit, there are some excellent first-aid kits available by mail order from wilderness supply catalogs. Good kits are also found in most drug stores. If money is a limited thing, you can put together your own by purchasing items one or two at a time until you feel you have what you need. This method is subject to procrastination, because it is too tempting to buy a six-pack of beer and think you will get the burn ointment. next week.

If you go into the city to sell some weaned pigs or a load of firewood, you might try the unfriendly high price surplus store. They may have an Army first-aid kit on which they failed to double the price last week.

Some fairly standard items for a first-aid kit are listed here:

1.   Roll of 1" wide gauze bandage
2.   Roll of 2" or 3" wide gauze bandage
3.   Sterile gauze pads in a couple of sizes
4.   Adhesive tape
5.   A box of adhesive bandages
6.   Burn ointment
7.   A box of cotton-tipped applicators
8.   A bottle of hydrogen peroxide
9.   A bottle of antiseptic
10. A pair of scissors (not the ones in the tool box or sewing kit).
11. A pair of tweezers
12. An X-acto knife
13. Poison Oak-Poison Ivy Lotion
14. Snake bite kit
15. Universal poison antidote

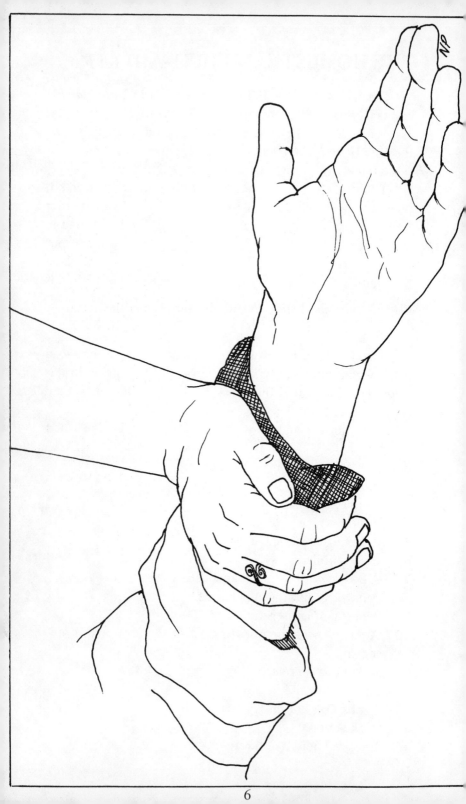

BLEEDING WOUNDS

Arterial bleeding, recognized by rhythmic beats, is one of the most serious emergencies. Immediately apply direct pressure to the wound. Obviously if you are down cutting firewood by the creek and someone is careless with the chain saw, you won't have a stash of certified sterile, hospital-quality dressings on hand. Don't hesitate to use your shirt or nearly anything else handy. Naturally, the cleaner the better. Apply direct, firm pressure to the wound, between it and the heart.

This is much like stopping a leak in the water line from the spring when you forget it's there and hit it with your grub hoe while digging a hole for the new outhouse.

It is possible to die within minutes from severe arterial bleeding. Do not waste time.

If direct pressure alone won't stop the bleeding, you can also apply pressure with a finger on the artery at pressure points as shown in the picture. Do this by forcing the artery against the bone with your finger.

You probably won't have our fine lucid text with you so you may want to practice locating those points on a friend (preferably opposite sex).

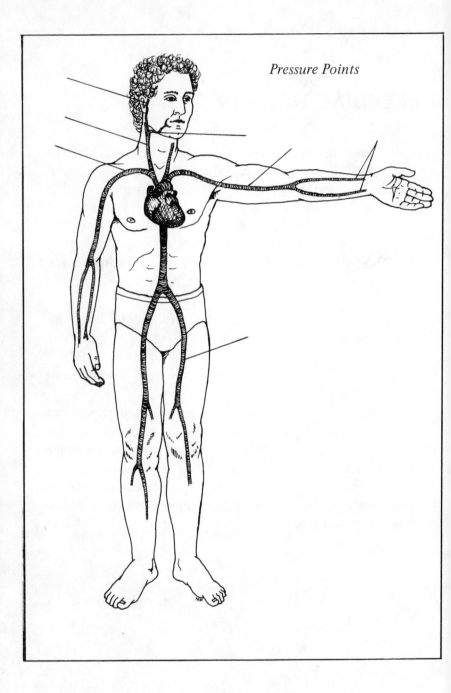

Pressure Points

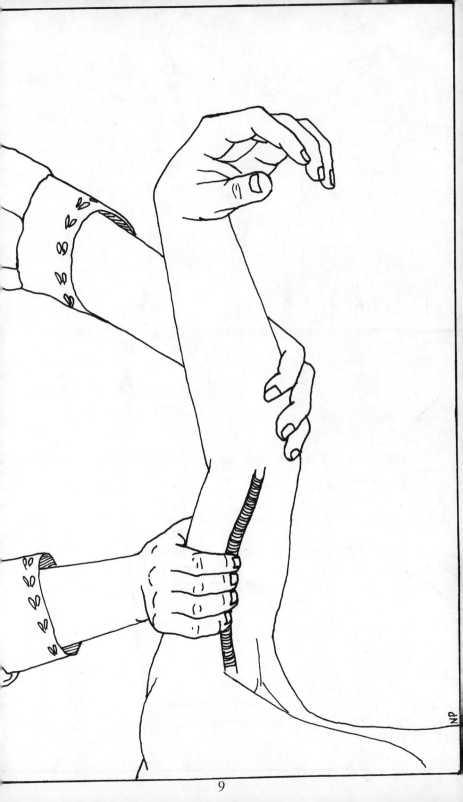

9

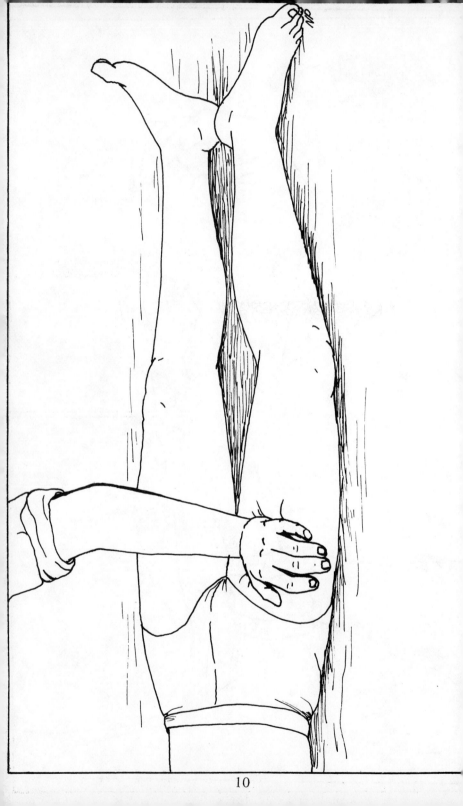

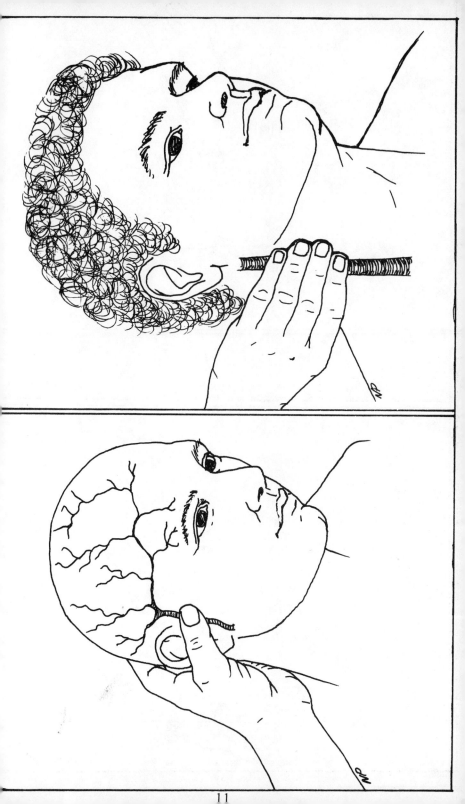

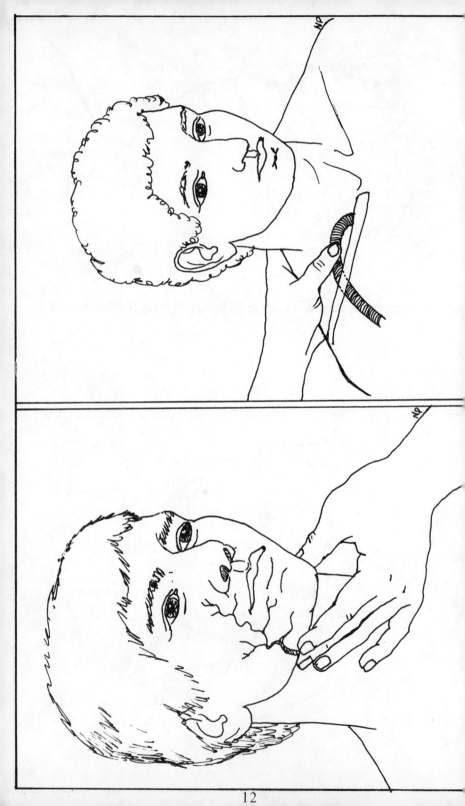

The tourniquet is the last refuge if direct pressure and pressure points don't stop the bleeding. But using a tourniquet may require surgery to forever eliminate another injury to that limb by amputating it. Most homesteaders deeply enjoy life, and would rather lose an arm than die.

A tourniquet may be a strip of cloth, a belt or a rag. Do not use a wire, cord or rope.

With a pad on top of the artery, pass the tourniquet twice around the limb above the wound. Twist the tourniquet until the bleeding stops, and then tie it.

Do not remove or loosen the tourniquet until surgery to the artery can be done. Death can result from tourniquet shock caused by alternate loosening and tightening. For later medical treatment, record the time the tourniquet was applied. As soon as bleeding has stopped treat for shock.

Remember: always apply pressure *above* the wound, between it and the heart. Otherwise it won't do any good.

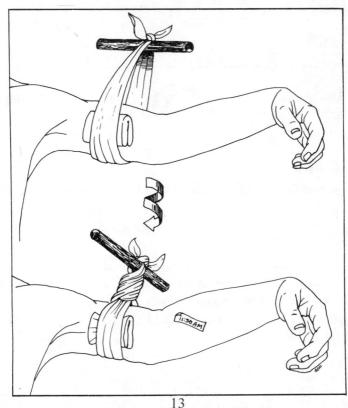

If the wound is less serious or if direct pressure or pressure points have controlled the bleeding, a pressure dressing of gauze or your clean shirt should be put on the wound.

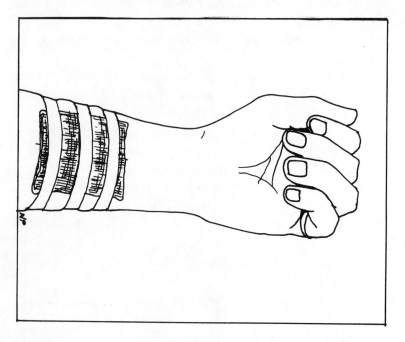

This should be held firmly by tape or strips of cloth and tied firmly. Tied too tightly, it may stop the flow of blood in the veins and increase blood pressure, causing more bleeding.

If necessary, the edges of the wound can be drawn together and held with pieces of tape.

Bleeding from the head or neck is treated much the same way, but care must be taken not to stop the flow of blood to the brain. This will cause unconsciousness and possibly death.

Less serious cuts may be treated by dousing them with an antiseptic and bandaging with Band-Aids or gauze and tape. If the cut is not serious, it is good to let it bleed a little. Bacteria carried by your pocket knife (or whatever made the cut) will flow out.

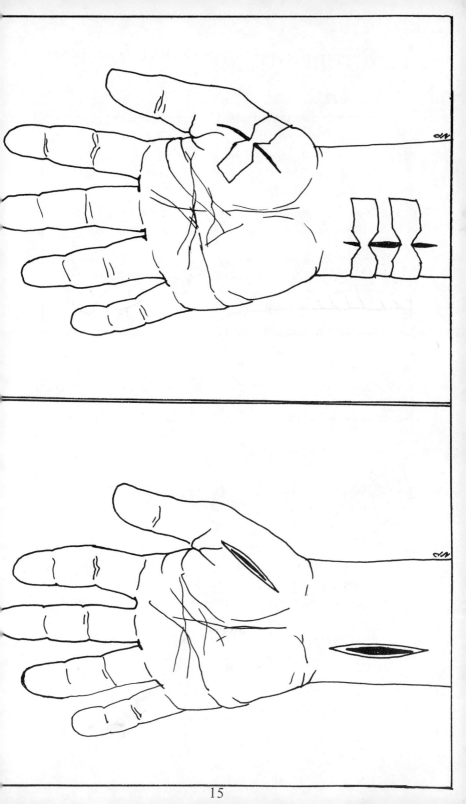

PUNCTURE WOUNDS

You may have left an old 2x6 laying on the ground from the barn you pulled down in order to build your house. You may have forgotten to pull the nails out of it. If you step on it in your haste to get plastic on your roof before a storm clears the next ridge, you'll probably have a puncture wound, as well as a mighty sore foot.

Go ahead, cuss, but remember to blame yourself.

First aid for this wound is to squeeze around the hole to

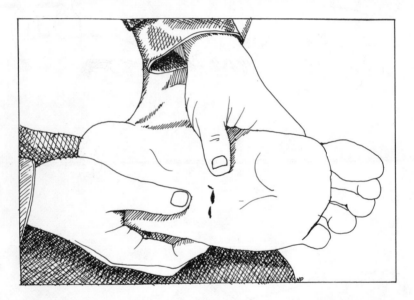

encourage the contaminated blood out, drench with iodine or hydrogen peroxide, and bandage. If you haven't had a recent tetanus shot, get one. This type of accident is perfect for getting tetanus bacteria into the flesh.

Splinters and deep knife wounds are treated similarly.

NOSE BLEEDS.

Nose bleed may sometimes be stopped by simple pressure with your thumbs against the upper lip just below the nose.

This will probably fix five year old Johnny's bloody nose when he comes flying over the creek bridge from the neighbors'. To treat a more serious nose bleed, place cotton in the victim's nostrils. A small amount should protrude from each nostril. Firmly squeeze the nostrils together with your thumb and finger for at least six minutes.

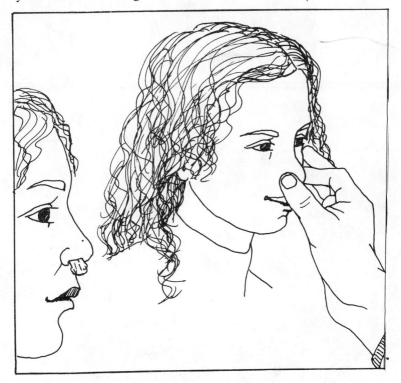

Put cold, wet towels over the face and nostrils. Gradually relieve pressure but leave the cotton inserted for several hours. If this doesn't stop the bleeding, or if it is recurrent, see a doctor.

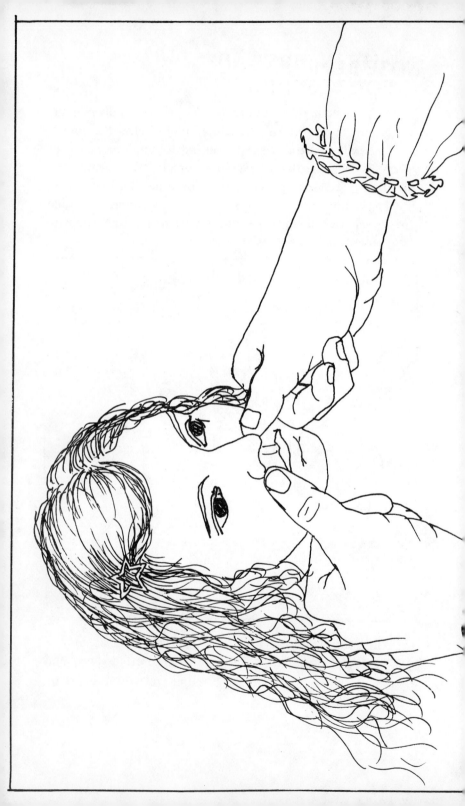

DON'TS IN FIRST-AID
FOR BLEEDING

1. Don't touch the wound with your fingers or anything else that might be contaminated.
2. Don't breath or cough on the wound.
3. Don't wash into a wound.
4. Don't disturb blood clots.
5. Don't use alcohol or other strong antiseptics on a wound near eyes or body openings.
6. Don't use cotton or tape directly on a wound.
7. Don't bandage too loosely or too tightly.

RESUSCITATION

Our bodies don't function long without air. Breathing can be stopped during unconsciousness, by something becoming stuck in the wind pipe or a combination of things. In the event that something is stuck in the throat, it is necessary to remove it before mouth-to-mouth breathing will work. The danger of diving into someone's throat to remove something is that whatever it is may be lodged further in the wind pipe. If the victim is a child hold him upside down and slap him sharply between the shoulder blades. If it is an adult, he may be laid face down on something with the head lower than the body and hit on the back.

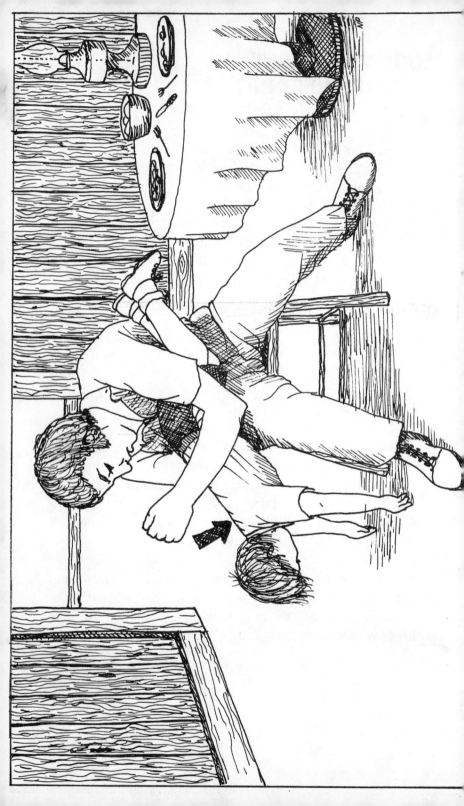

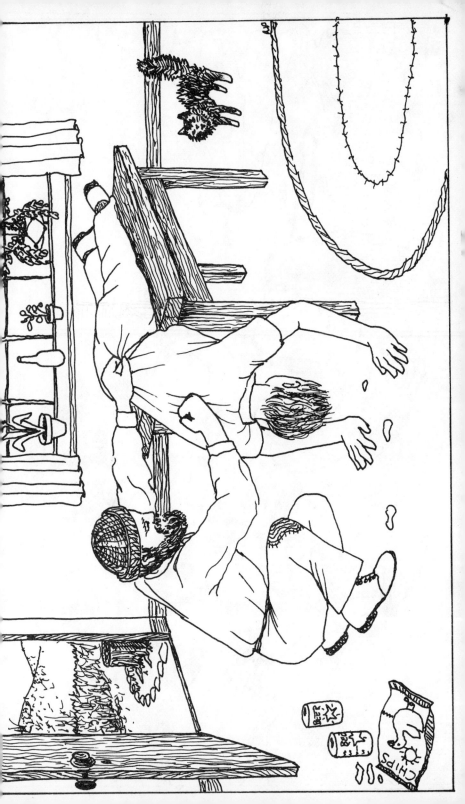

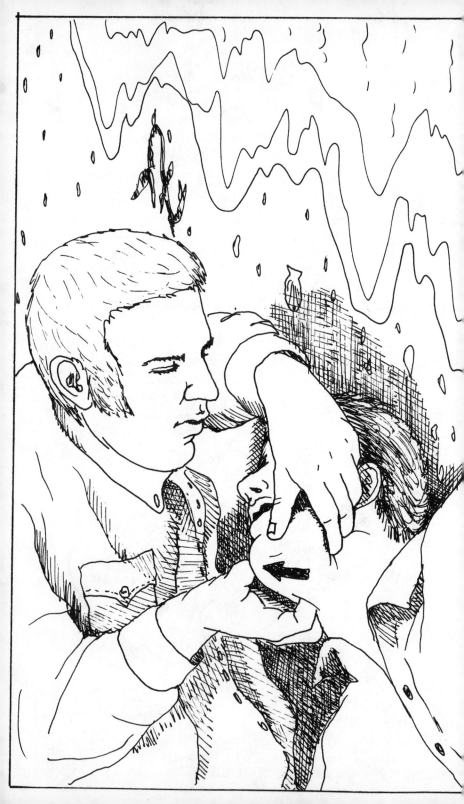

In most cases this will unstick whatever was stuck. If it doesn't, immediate medical aid should be sought. In an absolute emergency, where death will otherwise result, a hole may be cut in the throat below the adam's apple to get air into the wind pipe. This is a very dangerous operation and should be done by a doctor. Of course, if the victim dies first, a doctor won't help too much.

Sometimes vomit or mucus will clog the windpipe during unconsciousness. Lay the victim on his stomach with his head down to expel it from the throat. If a person is not breathing, do not lose any time in forcing air into his lungs. Anything over ten seconds to get a victim ready for resuscitation is too long.

Mouth-to-mouth breathing is the most effective, easiest to use resuscitation method. It requires no special equipment and gets more air into the victim's lungs faster than anything but a mechanical resuscitator. Although little skill is required, some practice with a suitable person may not be a bad way to learn the method in case you should ever need to use it. Could be fun, too.

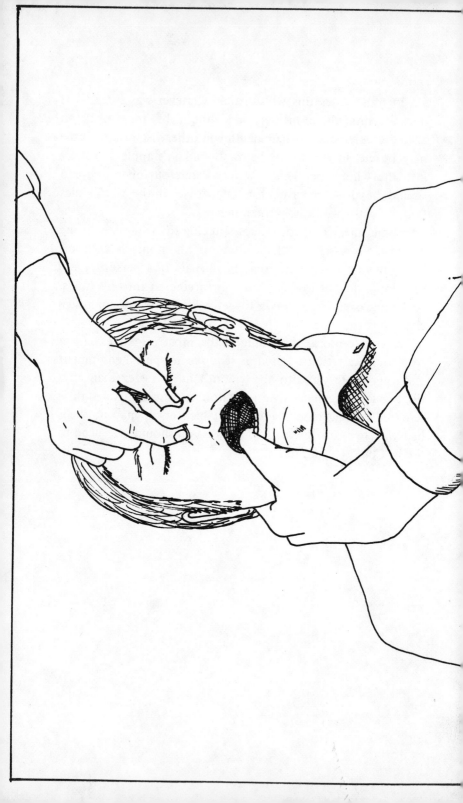

TREATMENT

1. The victim should be lying on his back.
2. Remove anything that may be in his mouth, also making sure the tongue is not covering the windpipe.
3. Tilt the victim's head back and pull the jaw up. This is important. The idea is to have as little resistance to the incoming air as possible.
4. Taking deep breaths, blow air. Blow vigorously for an adult, more gently for children. Blow into the victim's mouth, holding the nostrils closed. Use puffs from the checks for children under three years old.
5. When the victim's chest rises, remove your mouth to let him exhale.
6. After exhalation, repeat every two to five seconds until the victim's breathing is normal again.
7. Do not attempt to get water out of the lungs of a victim. Give mouth-to-mouth right away.

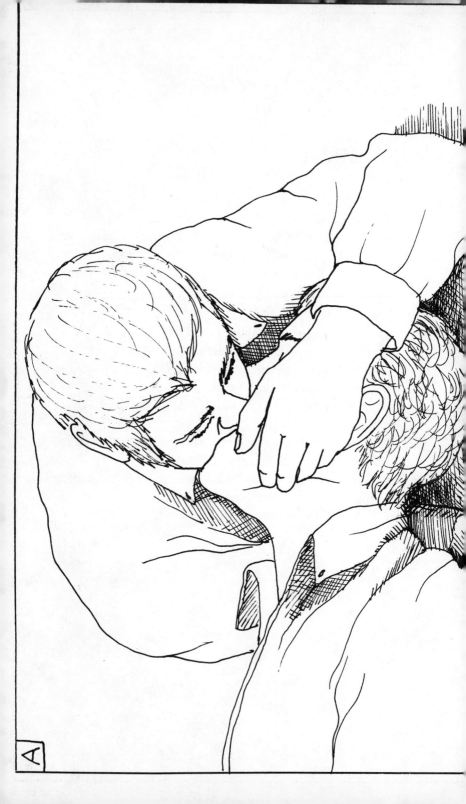

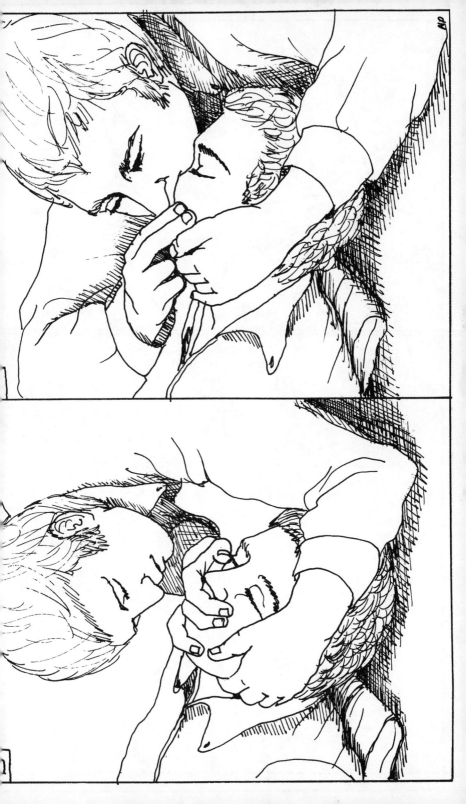

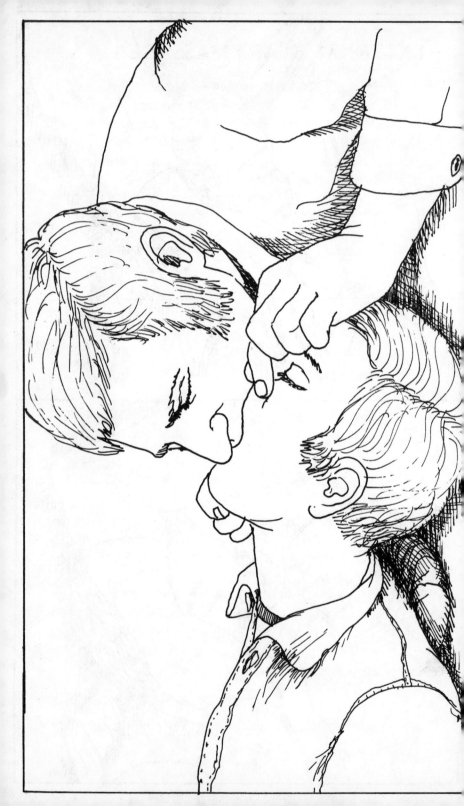

EXTERNAL HEART MASSAGE

If a victim's heart is found to be stopped or very weak, it will be necessary to use external heart massage. This is done by squeezing the heart between the breastbone and backbone. Lay the victim on his back on the floor or ground. Stand or kneel at right angles to the chest and give mouth-to-mouth breathing for several breaths.

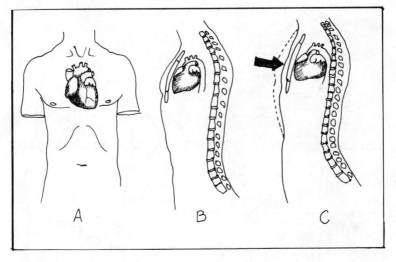

TREATMENT

1. Place your hands, one on top of the other on the lower part of the breastbone. Apply enough pressure to move the breast bone about two inches toward the spine. Too much pressure may break the ribs or damage heart muscle.
2. Relax and let the chest expand. Repeat rhythmically.
3. Someone else should be giving mouth-to-mouth breathing simultaneously. If there is no one available, you may stop every one-half minute to give mouth-to-mouth for four or five deep breaths.

Compressing the heart this way forces blood from the heart to the arteries. It's like priming the pump in the south pasture.

29

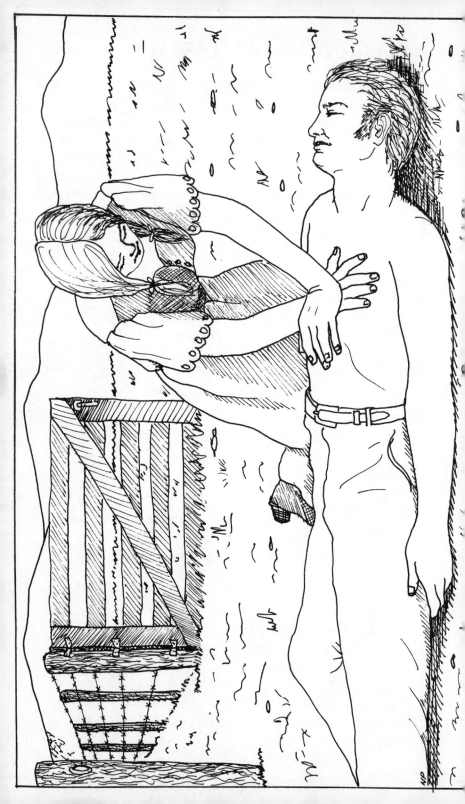

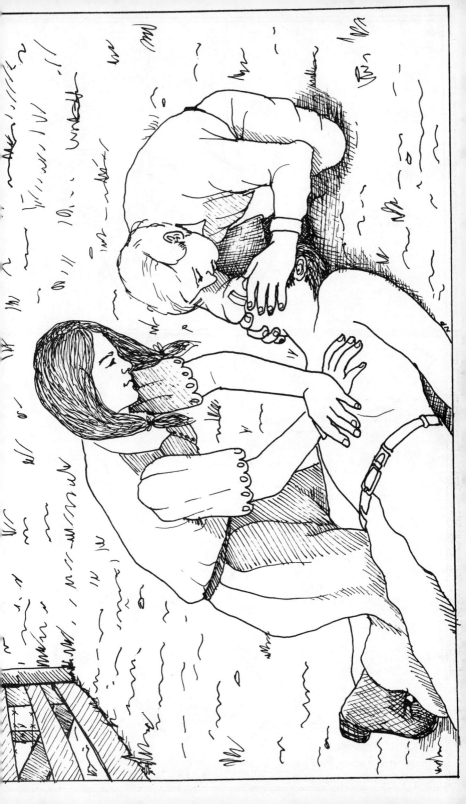

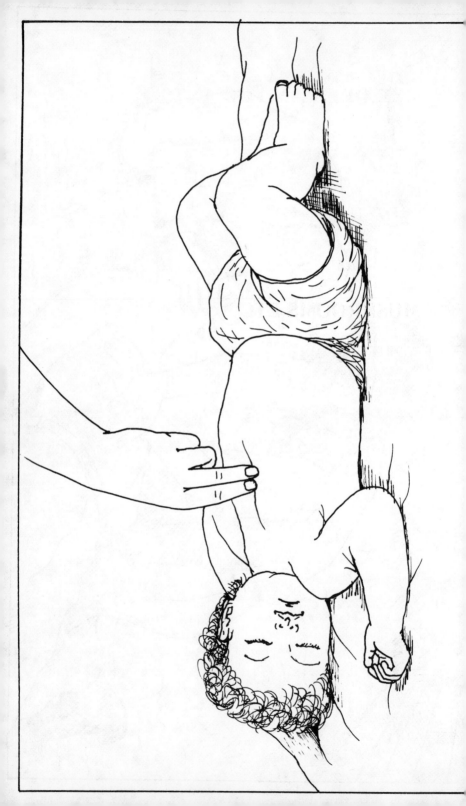

CHILDREN AND INFANTS

External heart massage for children is the same as adults, using much less pressure. For babies, only very moderate pressure with the finger tips should be used. Their hearts may be easily damaged.

MUSHROOMS ETC

The homestead is often abundant with wild plants which are great for smoking, making salads, or brewing up an excellent tea. However, it is very important to carefully identify any wild plants before making up a salad from greens growing in the meadows or down by the creek. Not long ago, the neighbor down the road had a terrifying experience. He had been reading an obscure herbal book while snowed in for a few days. When the snow melted he thought he recognized one of the plants in the book and, after cutting a little firewood, he brought the plant home with him. That was at lunch time. He made a tea from the plant and wasn't seen again until a search party located him about four A.M. the next morning. He was sitting on an old fir stump on the Walsh place entertaining some Leprechauns he had met there. As you can see from the terrible experience of neighbor John, it is important that you take every precaution and be certain of the identity of plants and herbs before bringing them into the kitchen. Just because goats find poison oak a savory delight doesn't mean it would make a particularly good tea or whatever.

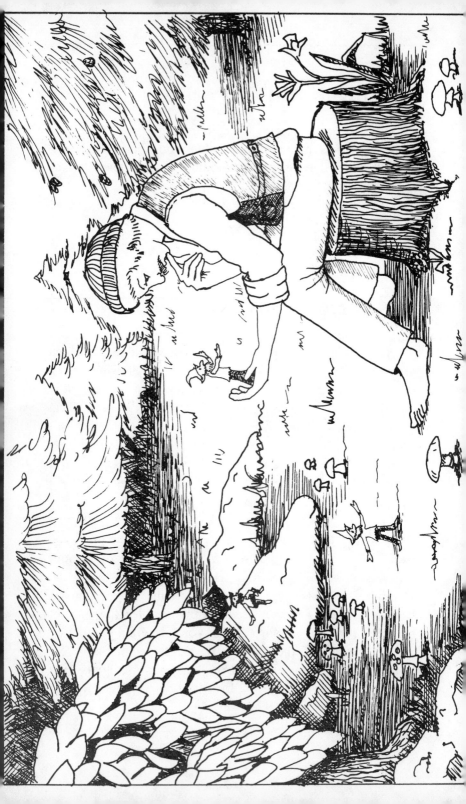

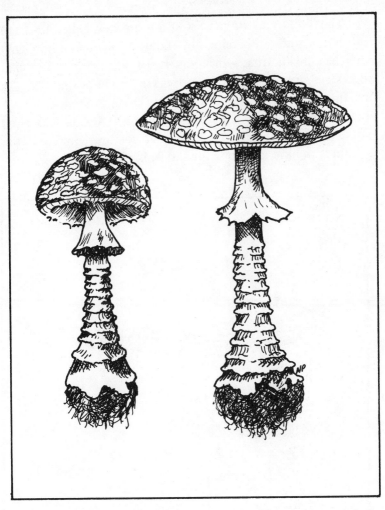

The classic of wild plant hassles is the mushroom. It is the most tempting bounty in nature's store of wild foods. Some species are very poisonous, however. Many times local legend may be the best way to learn which are what. It may be wise to hunt mushrooms with the old lady down the road who grew up picking mushrooms. Her age is some judgment of her knack for mushroom identity.

The most feared is a group of mushrooms that produces a poison that liquifies tissue cells in the body, particularly the red blood cells. These are protoplasmic poisons. Named after the most common species, they are commonly called Amanita mushrooms.

35

The symptoms of these poisons are delayed from 10 to 20 hours and are commonly fatal. Violent vomiting and diarrhea are the first symptoms. If the poisoning isn't fatal in this stage, it progressively destroys vital body organs. There is no first-aid for this type of poisoning except to induce vomiting if the victim or suspected victim isn't already, and treat for shock. Immediate medical attention is required if the victim is to have any hope for survival.

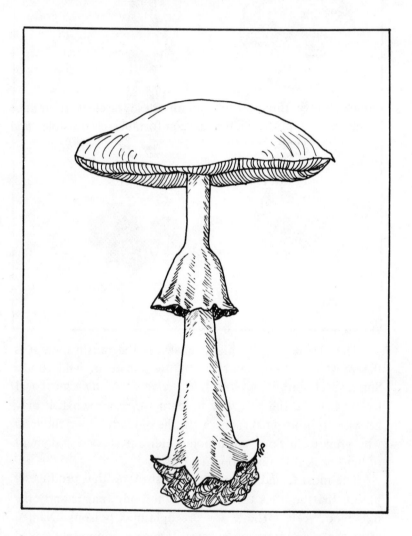

The muscarine group of mushrooms produces a poison that is toxic to the nerves. Some of the symptoms are similar to Amanita Poisoning; but they appear in 15 to 30 minutes. Besides vomiting and diarrhea, the victim begins to sweat and salivate heavily. Visual disturbances, low pulse, low blood pressure and asthmatic breathing are other symptoms.

Besides these unpleasant symptoms, and an awful mess in the outhouse, muscarine poisoning rarely has any more serious affects. Treatment is the same as for Amanita poisons.

Several other species produce poisons which are not as serious unless large quantities are consumed. At least a couple of species are known to produce an alcohol-like intoxication and some to cause folks to hallucinate or do some strange things. First aid in these cases is to induce vomiting, keep the victim as comfortable as possible, and give him whatever other fluids and foods he can hold down.

It is important to emphasize again, though, that mushroom poisoning, especially since identification by the unskilled is rarely accurate, should be treated as a very serious problem.

FOOD POISONS

In many ways the present generation of homesteaders has it much better than our grandparents did. One of these is the advantage of having a better understanding of the unseen world of bacteria.

Bacteria turns the manure pile to good garden compost, gets the mash barrel fermenting and makes good wine for us, but some of the omnipresent little guys can devastate the homestead family if they get out of hand in the kitchen.

Clostridium botulinum bacteria is common in any farm environment. It is the bacteria which causes the most serious type of food poisoning called botulism. It is always present to some extent in vegetables, as it is an anerobic bacteria. Bacteria find an ideal environment in improperly canned vegetables, especially green beans. The clostridium botulinum thrives and multiplies here, producing a strong toxic to the human nervous system. Death occurs from strangulation or heart failure in most of the untreated cases.

Identifying botulism is often difficult because the symptoms may not appear for a day or two after contaminated food has been eaten. Besides upset stomach, the victim of botulism will experience dim vision, double vision and paralysis of the throat muscles, causing difficulty with talking and choking when trying to swallow.

Beyond first aid treatment for the obvious symptoms while *en route to the hospital* there is no effective treatment other than medically administered antitoxin. Early diagnosis and treatment is essential as the antitoxin will only halt more damage to the nervous system. It will not reverse damage already done.

Careful canning and cooking practices have virtually eliminated botulism poisoning cases. All canned foods should be well cooked before eating and any suspicious appearing canned goods should be used on the compost pile only.

STAPHYLOCOCCIC FOOD POISONING

Staphylococcus bacteria thrive in meats, dairy products and baked foods when the refrigerator breaks down or the food is left on the table too long and becomes warm. These bacteria produce a toxin which is unaffected by subsequent cooking or heating and cause violent nausea, vomiting and diarrhea. If you have ever witnessed five adults and a couple of children to one outhouse all affected simultaneously, you fully understand the seriousness of this condition.

Although an otherwise healthy person rarely experiences any lasting effects, staphylococcic poisoning often inspires one to wish that he would die or at least to plead "O Lord, if you get me through this one, I'll get through the next one myself".

First aid again can only be for the symptoms. In case of severe poisoning, shock sometimes results. The vomiting and diarrhea in themselves, though, are the best first aid as they expel the toxin from the body.

SALMONELLA POISONING

Salmonella group of bacteria contaminate the same group of food as staphylococcus bacteria, but are spread by a carrier and proliferate where unsanitary conditions occur. The carrier may be a person, insects or rodents. Cooking and refrigeration do not affect these bacteria. They mostly remain dormant until they enter the human intestinal tract.

Poorly built outhouses that don't exclude common rodents and insects, improper disposal of grey water and contamination of drinking water from leeching are conducive to a good out-break of Salmonella poisoning.

Symptoms are stomach cramps, nausea and diarrhea. Treatment is limited to making the victim as comfortable as possible. If diarrhea is too severe, a little paragoric may be used.

CHEMICAL POISONING

Leaving the asphalt and concrete behind for clean air in the mountains and fresh food from the garden doesn't guarantee the homestead family immunity from the harsh reality of poisoning. Small children are eager to learn about their world, usually through their mouths. Medicine chests, kitchen cabinets and tool sheds are particularly enchanting to the small folks eager to react with their environment and to learn of the many mysteries that live there.

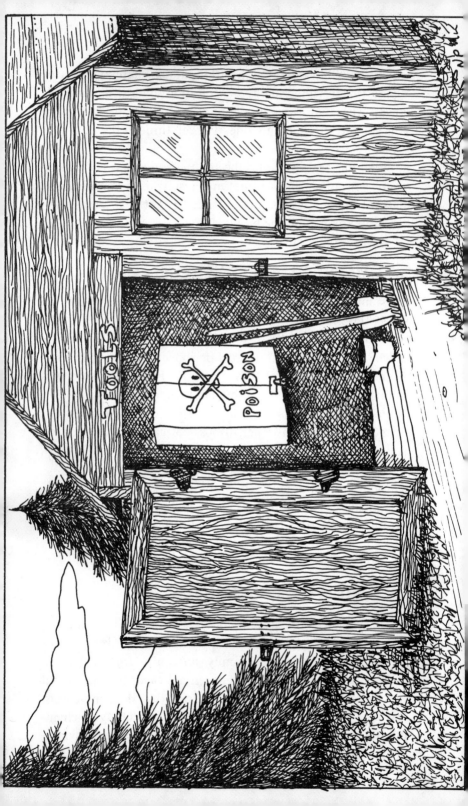

Many items and chemicals around the homestead, including things that aren't labeled poison, can cause death or serious injury if they are swallowed by children. Some substances that are not really considered poisonous can cause poisoning if large quantities are taken.

Aspirin, prescription medicines, tonics and laxatives are among these. Some awareness of these dangers and securing all potentially dangerous substances beyond the reach of little people may avert a tragedy.

Always keep medicines, veterinary supplies, and other dangerous or poisonous substances in a place that children cannot get to and preferably in a cabinet that can be locked. Avoid storing these items in anything other than their original containers. If you have shared a large quantity purchase with a neighbor and use glass jars for lye or a syrup can for kerosene for the aladdin lamp, make certain these containers are conspicuously relabeled.

IMPORTANT DON'TS
IN POISONING

1. Don't waste time by going to the neighbors to use the phone to call for help until you have diluted the poison and washed it out.
2. Don't force fluids into an unconscious or very drowsy poisoning victim.
3. Don't try to cause vomiting if the poison is kerosene, gasoline or other petroleum product; or if the poison is a strong acid or alkali.
4. Don't wait for symptoms of poisoning to appear. Give immediate first aid and get the victim to medical help.

SYMPTOMS OF POISONING

If Johnny comes into the house after being out in the yard for some time with the home liniment on his breath or red paint around his mouth, it is obvious that he may have swallowed something that could be dangerous. Other symptoms may be more subtle. Here is a list of the more common:

1. Vomiting and pain or burning in the mouth, throat, and stomach.
2. Convulsions, restlessness, excitement, or irritability.
3. Irregular breathing which may be either weak and slow or deep and rapid.
4. Drowsiness, confusion and slurred speech.
5. Burns or discoloration around the mouth, tongue or chin.
6. Breath odor.
7. Unconsciousness.

What is done in the first few minutes after a victim has swallowed a poison may mean the difference between a funeral service and long and happy life. A poison must be diluted, washed out of the stomach or neutralized as quickly as possible to prevent irreparable damage to vital organs.

FIRST-AID FOR POISONING

1. Give large amounts of warm soapy water, or water with either a tablespoon full of baking soda or salt or just plain water or milk if the above aren't available. If the poison is known and an antidote is on the label use it if it is immediately available.
2. Induce vomiting to empty the stomach only if the poison is not a petroleum product, or an acid or alkali. (Breath odor will indicate a petroleum poisoning, burns on lips, chin and in the mouth will indicate an acid or alkali.) Vomiting may be induced in other cases by tickling the back of the throat with your finger. If the victim is a child, hold him across your lap with his head lower than his body.

42

3. If your first aid kit contains activated charcoal or prepared universal antidote for poisoning, administer it at this time. If not, use crumpled up burned toast, milk of magnesia, egg whites in milk and strong tea or large amounts of water if nothing else is available.

4. Repeat the above steps after a few minutes. Do this several times until the vomit is clear, then add egg whites or flour in water. Watch the victim carefully for signs of shock and failure to breathe.

5. Treat for shock and give mouth-to-mouth breathing if and as required.

6. Give victim hot tea or coffee if he is conscious.

7. Get victim to hospital or clinic. If possible, take the poison container as well as a sample of the vomited matter with you to aid the doctor in identifying the poison.

TREATMENT OF
SPECIFIC POISONS

When you know for sure what the poisoning agent is, more specific first aid can be given. Many poisons are common petroleum products, strong acids and alkalies.

COMMON PETROLEUM PRODUCTS

1. Gasoline   4. Paint Thinners   7. Lighter Fluid
2. Kerosene   5. Cleaning Solvent   8. Naptha
3. Diesel Oil   6. Benzene   9. Oils

Do not induce vomiting if any of these things have been swallowed. These could be the most dangerous to the homestead family as there is no first aid. Immediate hospitalization is necessary. Avoid using petroleum based chemicals

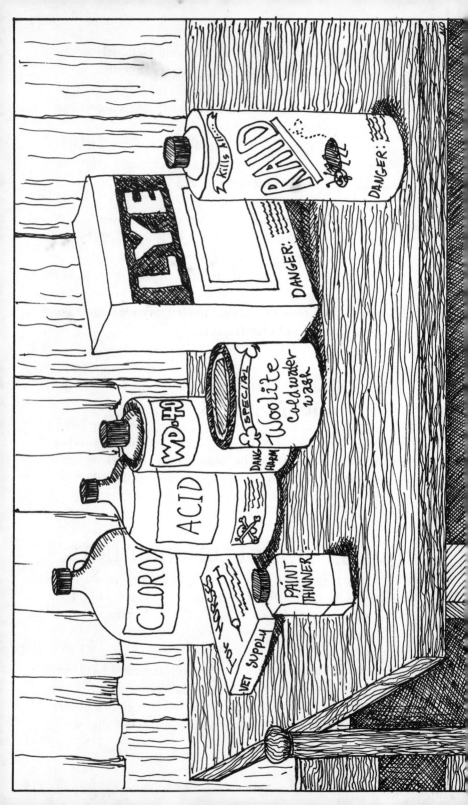

whenever possible, store them very carefully and never keep petroleum products in food containers.

Wine jugs, fruit jars and pop bottles are usually the most readily available containers for kerosene, paint thinner, etc., but get metal containers for these.

COMMON ACIDS

1. Sulfuric Acids – used in car batteries.
2. Hydrochloric Acid – used in barn and household disinfectants and in some veterinary supplies.
3. Oxalic Acid – used in cleaning solution and making dyes.
4. Creaol or Creosote – used in veterinary medicine, wood preservatives and disinfectants.

Do not induce vomiting if any of the above or other acids have been swallowed. Give the victim, (except for carbolic acid or creosol poisoning) the prepared universal antidote, or baking soda dissolved in water, or milk of magnesia. The idea here is to neutralize the acid without trying to make the victim vomit. The strain of vomiting can cause rupture of vital organs, that may have been damaged by the acids swallowed. If vomiting can't be helped, try to keep the victim from straining.

CARBOLIC ACID OR CREOSOL

Carbolic Acid or creosol poisoning will produce a distinctive odor on the breath and in vomited matter. Whiskey, wine, grain alcohol are specific neutralizing agents for these acids and should be given liberally to the victim of this type of poisoning. If you give him enough he may not even care if he is sick or not. If no alcohol is available as is usually the case on any good Christian Homestead (it seems to evaporate from the stoppered bottle), give egg whites beaten up in water or soapy water. The victim should now be made to vomit and empty the stomach. Follow this with milk, milk with eggs beaten up in it (egg nog if you just happen to have made a batch) and/or tea to soothe the stomach.

For external treatment of acid burns use baking soda, but not in the eyes.

Even if the victim seems comfortable after first aid treatment he should be examined by a doctor.

CORROSIVE ALKALIES

These poisons may be among the most hazardous, as they are commonly found in large quantities on the homestead. Some of them are as follows. *Ammonia* is used in cleaners for the house and the barn as well as for fertilizer. (Organic farming will eliminate that danger.) *Lime* is used in mortar for masonry work, for sweetening acid soil in the garden and to disguise the smell in the outhouse. *Potash* is also common as a fertilizer. *Lye* and *Caustic Soda* are used in making soap.

Again vomiting may further damage internal organs and should not be induced. If a corrosive alkali has been swallowed give the victim vinegar and water or large quantities of lemon or orange juice. These will neutralize the alkali. Follow with milk, milk and eggs, vegetable oil or flour and water to coat and protect the stomach.

NOTE

A universal antidote may be made up and kept in the first aid kit. If there are little folks around, this might be a good idea. The recipe is two parts of activated charcoal, one part magnesium oxide and one part tannic acid.

46

METAL COMPOUND POISONING

Many poisonous metal compounds may be part of homestead life. Arsenic copper and mercury are common in rat and mice poisons, and plant and animal sprays. Lead is found in paint, zinc is used in weed killers and in the shot in welding and soldering.

Treatment is to dilute and wash out as in the basic first aid for poisoning given previously. (Steps one thru seven.)

WOOD ALCOHOL

Alcohol fuels, rubbing alcohol, some anti-freeze solutions and lacquer thinner — treat as above in basic first aid for poison and administer Epsom Salt in water.

STRYCHNINE

Strychnine is found in many rat poisons, some laxatives and street produced drugs. Strychnine poisoning can cause cessation of breathing, violent convulsions. It is essential that the victim is treated before these symptoms appear. Dilute and wash out the poison and give the universal antidote or iodine diluted in water or very strong tea. DO NOT GIVE COFFEE. Get the victim to medical help immediately. If breathing stops, give mouth-to-mouth.

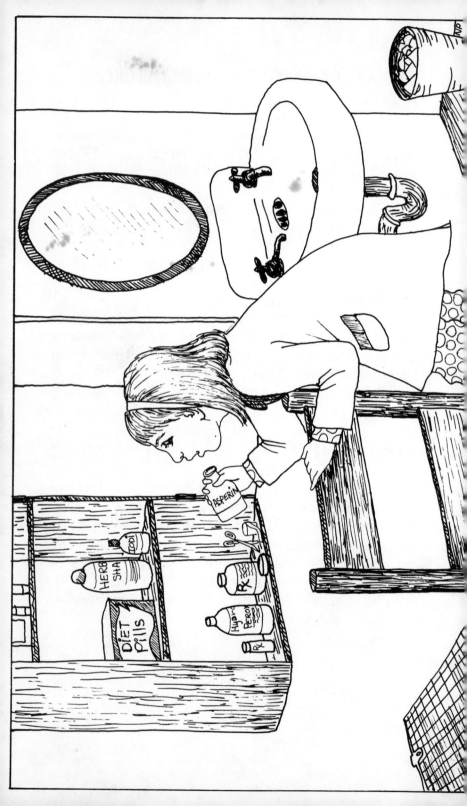

ASPIRIN POISONING

Aspirin can be a dangerous drug if a child takes an entire bottle. Many flavored aspirins are marketed for children to increase sales and to induce the child to take them. This may be great for the drug manufacturers but the child may conclude that if they taste good and mommy wants him to take one occasionally that a whole bottle may be better. It is probably best if flavored aspirin are not used. A standard aspirin tablet may be sliced into quarters and given to the kids if it is necessary. And these we keep locked in the medicine chest. Right?

Symptoms of aspirin poisoning may not occur for from several hours to a day. If a possible aspirin poisoning is detected, do not wait for symptoms to appear, but get treatment right away.

The first physical symptom is rapid and deep breathing, irritability and restlessness. By this time, internal chemistry is doing some damage on other body organs that can be dangerous or even fatal. In an advanced condition it may cause bleeding in the stomach and vomiting up blood.

TREATMENT

1. If aspirin poisoning is discovered soon after it has happened, the stomach should be emptied and washed repeatedly by inducing vomiting with a finger tickling the back of the throat and giving large amounts of water.
2. If any symptoms have begun to appear, immediate hospitalization is necessary, no first aid techniques will help. Treat as for shock and give mouth-to-mouth breathing.

BURNS

Homesteads, by nature, offer a plethora of burn hassels. Wood heat stoves, kerosene lamps, gas cook stoves, cooking on open fire and heating water on the stove are things most common to country life. Burns can be as simple as sunburn from too much time at the swimming hole, or grabbing the hot muffler of the chain saw, or from the still blowing up in the middle of a special run for the Sunday afternoon pot luck lunch and hoe down. Not only is it anguish to lose your still, but the resulting burns can be very painful. Curiosity about matches and fire, and the desire to help with the summer canning and cook-out makes the children on the homestead particularly likely to be burned. Good consciousness of burn and fire dangers and supervised experience of fire and heat by the kids go a long way in preventing these accidents.

Burns are classed medically by degree, from first to fourth according to the depth of the burn. First degree is like a cigarette burn on the finger; fourth degree is like falling in the camp fire. First aid for burns is limited and the degree of burn is not important to first aid treatment except that some minor first and second degree burns may not require the whole family getting in the Chevy flatbed and heading for town. They may be taken care of at home with some knowledge of burn treatment.

First degree burns are superficial burns to the skin. They are characterized by local reddening of the area burned. Sunburns are usually in this catagory but can sometimes be second degree.

Picking up a hot horseshoe not long out of the forge or grabbing the coffee pot on the Ashley when it's too hot usually produces our regular garden variety second degree burn, which is characterized by blisters.

TREATMENT

1. The usual response to a burn is to get it in the creek or other cold water. Soak the burn or keep covering it with clean towels soaked in ice cold water. Baking soda may be used in the soak water.
2. The cold water will do much to reduce the pain. If the burn has not charred the skin you should then use a good non-greasy, antiseptic burn ointment on the skin. The ointment will prevent infection and keep the skin from drying and cracking. A good burn ointment will have some local anesthetic in it which will help ease the pain.
3. Blisters on a second degree burn may be opened to drain with a flamed needle or knife point. Apply an antiseptic to the hole and cover with a sterile dressing.

TREATMENT OF SERIOUS BURNS

Burns of third or fourth degree need immediate medical attention. First aid is limited to treatment for shock, gentle removal of any clothing stuck to the burn, and covering the burn with sterile gauze or clean pieces of bed sheet or something similar. Give the victim as much water or other fluids as he can take.

SUNBURN

Severe sunburns should have the same medical attention as any other serious burns. Otherwise, gently apply a sunburn ointment, baby oil or olive oil. Some iodine solution in the oil may be helpful as well. Cover any blistered areas as above and again give the victim large amounts of fluids.

SUNSTROKE

Summer haying, barn building and septic tank digging are things that should always be done in the cool hours of the day during summer. Kicking back in the afternoon with some cold homebrew, or lemonade (and talking to the herb garden) is the best prevention for sunstroke. Sunstroke (heat stroke is the same) generally occurs while working in high temperature and high humidity conditions. Perhaps this is why the mountain distiller prefers to work at night. The underlying cause is the stopping of sweating which is the human radiator. The common symptoms are collapse, flushed skin and very hot and dry skin. This condition can be very dangerous and should receive immediate medical attention.

IN THE MEANTIME

1. Get the victim into the coldest water possible even using ice, if it is available.
2. After a few minutes, the victim's temperature should be down to a hundred degrees. He may be removed from the water and wrapped in cold, wet sheets. If the body temperature should rise again, put him back in the water.
3. If immersion in cold water is impossible, do anything imaginable to cool the body down. Lying under a sprinkler should help. If there is no sprinkler, only cold beer, be sure to charge the victim after he recovers.
4. If an enema apparatus is available, administer an ice water enema to the victim. This is said to be a very effective way in lowering body temperature. It might also reward the rescuer with a kick in the head, though, so be careful.

HEAT EXHAUSTION

Heat exhaustion is a less serious reaction to environment stress by the hot sun. Fainting, weakness, headache, vomiting, dizziness, pale skin, heavy sweating and weak pulse are some of the usual symptoms. Note that sweating is present during heat exhaustion but note also the dry skin in the more serious stroke condition.

1. Lay the victim on his back in a cool place and loosen or remove his clothing. Especially get heavy, heat retaining Levi's off.
2. Give the victim doses of salt solution of one teaspoon of salt to a glass of water.
3. Follow with coffee, tea or other stimulants.

HEAT CRAMPS

Sometimes stomach cramps will occur when a large amount of water is consumed during high temperatures and the lost body salts are not replaced. Give the victim salt water as above or salt tablets. Massage the stomach muscles to relieve the cramps. It is best not to give salt or tablets with very cold water. Warmer water will have less shock to the system.

During summer months it is a good program to keep a jar of salt tablets on the kitchen table. Like other animals, our bodies will trigger a conscious desire for salt when it is needed.

53

CHEMICAL BURNS

Battery acid, creosote for fence posts, lye for soap making, gasoline and kerosene are some common homestead chemicals that can cause burns. Eyes are especially sensitive and vulnerable to these types of burns.

TREATING CHEMICAL BURNS IN THE EYES

1. Lay the victim down and wash the eye with water from a cup or glass for several minutes by holding the eyelid open. Tilt the victim's head so the rinse will run over the eye and out the corner easily.
2. Cover the eye with a sterile gauze pad or clean cloth held tightly in place and get medical attention if the burn is serious.

CHEMICAL BURNS TO THE SKIN

1. Remove any clothing that has the chemical on it.
2. Wash the area with water and treat as for other burns.

FROSTBITE

Winter on many homesteads poses the additional problem of frostbite. Usually the extremities of the body, the ears, face, fingers, toes and feet are commonly affected. Frostbite is the freezing and destroying of living tissue just as in a burn.

Symptoms of frostbite in its early stages are reddening of the skin, pain and numbness and a tingling sensation. As frostbite progresses, the skin becomes white, the area burns and itches and there is a loss of sensation in the frostbitten area.

FIRST-AID

1. If outdoors, press the frostbitten area against a warm part of the body and cover with wool or other cloth.
2. Get the victim into the kitchen with a warm fire and give him hot coffee or soup as soon as possible.
3. Thaw the affected area by immersing in water, NO WARMER THAN BODY TEMPERATURE, or wrap the area in a warm blanket.
4. Using a dry towel, massage gently toward the frozen area. Do not massage the frozen area directly.

Frostbite occurs quickly and is almost unnoticed when it is occuring, especially if you are very young and busy making a snowman or sliding down the road on an old sled. Be sure the children are dressed warmly and get them in the house for hot chocolate every hour or so.

CHILDHOOD ACCIDENTS AND ILLNESSES

The animals on our homestead have their young routinely scorning any interference by us, and they grow to maturity without incident. The only time the goats have been to the vet have been when we have polluted their environment with a piece of barbed wire left where it caught a low hanging udder, and a rusty nail that got imbedded in a young hoof. We give them a shot of home grown apple cider vinegar with their evening hay and they stay disgustingly healthy.

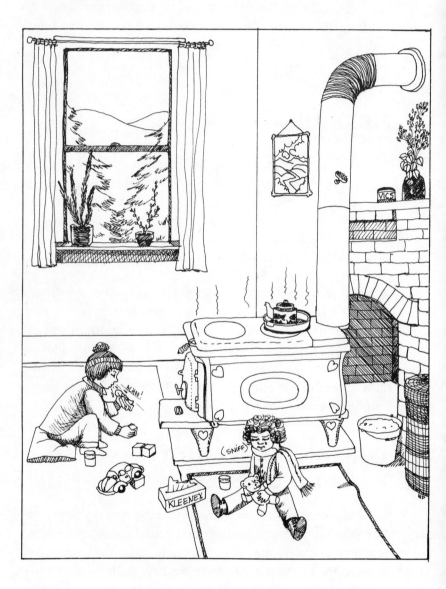

The young of the homestead family of man are a different story. They are susceptible to a hundred diseases and prone to all kinds of accidents. Fortunately, living in the country with clean air, garden vegetables and fresh milk makes tougher babies and most diseases and accidents are mild and over with soon. This section is to help you with some suggestions for taking care of the common childhood hassles until you can get medical attention.

Medical facilities and immunization clinics for children are often available free through county, state and federal programs. If you have small folks, don't wait until you need medical attention but investigate these services as soon as you arrive in the area.

It can be very frustrating to rush one of the kids to the hospital after falling on his head from a tree only to be told that they cannot treat him without proof of medical insurance or payment in cash. It would be a good idea to check into some type of health insurance as cash isn't always around when you need it.

COLDS

Most colds the small folks have will be mild ones if the kids are generally healthy and easily cared for at home. Confinement to bed is usually difficult and not necessary if they are not too sick and don't want to be. They should be dressed warmly and the fire stoked up enough to keep the house moderately warm.

Colds are almost impossible to prevent, especially if there are kids in that hot bed of potent disease germs, the public school. A good diet with a lot of natural vitamins, a lot of time outside doing chores and playing, and plenty of sleep in a moderately cool draft-free room will sure help, though. Colds are caused by a virus so small that it isn't visible even under many microscopes but it does need low body resistance to really get going good and make life seem downright disagreeable.

If there is a baby on the homestead every precaution should be taken to prevent his exposure to cold germs, especially during the first year.

Like adults the kids need plenty of juice with a lot of vitamin C, herb teas, hot honey with lemon juice and a touch of brandy for coughs. Given with plenty of love these will get them back to good health soon.

You can relieve the stuffed up nose in children too young to blow their nose with a nasal syringe, which might be a good item to have in the first aid kit. Depress the bulb of the syringe forcing the air from it, place the tip in the child's nostril and release the bulb. This will draw the mucus from the nose. Repeat gently until the nose is clear. In a severe case of congestion always consult a doctor. Nose drops made for children may be used on older children (check for specific age on the label) but only under a doctor's direction for younger children.

BRONCHITIS, PNEUMONIA

Bronchitis can be a simple chest cold and treated pretty much the same as a head cold, or it can be the beginning of a serious case of pneumonia. The child should be watched carefully. If fever over 101 degrees develops, or if his cough becomes serious, medical help should be sought. If you are lucky, your community may have a doctor who makes house calls.

EARACHE

An ear infection sometimes accompanies a cold. If the child is over two years old, he will be able to tell you he has an earache. If he is too young to communicate verbally he will probably pull at the sore ear while yelling his head off. Beyond putting a loose cotton plug in the ear, there is little that can be done at home and early medical treatment should be sought.

CROUP

Croup is a dry, harsh cough with difficult breathing. It is a very serious condition and should have medical attention as quickly as possible. A vaporizer, if you have electricity, will give some relief. If nothing else, warm steamy wet towels held over the nose and throat will help.

CONVULSIONS

Children will sometimes have convulsions at the beginning of a cold or the onset of a fever. Convulsions are not necessarily a sign of a more serious condition but a medical opinion should be sought if they are recurrent. Try to get the child on a bed or something soft; on the floor with a pillow under his head is better than nothing. Put something soft such as a clean cotton sock or a wadded piece of cloth in his mouth so he won't bite his tongue. His clothes should be removed if possible, or at least enough to prevent choking or breaking a bone from being twisted. If he is in bed, watch that he doesn't fall off and try to keep him on his side so that if he vomits he will not choke. Ice packs on the head and the back of the neck, and rinsing with a rag dipped in cool water will also help. Do not put the child in a bathtub, as he can easily hurt himself or even drown if he gets out of control. Fortunately, convulsions are short lived.

HEAD INJURIES

The present survival of our species never ceases to amaze; it seems the only way kids learn their limitations is to fall on their heads a few times and the homestead presents un-

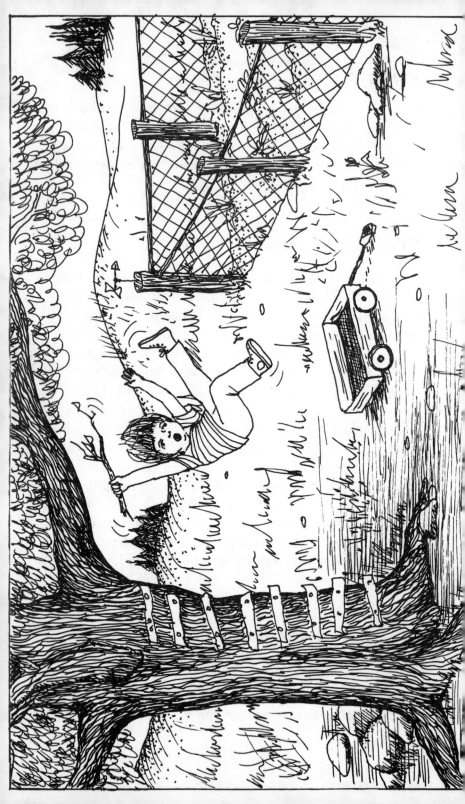

limited opportunities for self destruction in this fashion.

Most of the time when one of the flock falls from his perilous perch on the limb of the oak tree in the pasture, his cry brings mom running from the breakfast dishes to scoop the injured from the ground, and a tender kiss on the forehead makes everything better.

Remember that a child's head is not nearly as hard as it should probably be or even seems to be when they jump up in your lap and hit your nose with it. The majority of childhood accidents are the bump-on-the-head variety. A serious fall can cause concussion or contusion with or without a fracture to the skull. In any serious head injury to a child, it is best to do nothing until you are sure of the type and severity of the injury.

TREATMENT

1. Lay the child on his back and treat for shock, but do not try to force liquids into him if he is not fully conscious.
2. If possible, do not move the child while awaiting a doctor. If he must be moved, use a stretcher. Lay him on his back and move him very carefully and gently.
3. While awaiting medical help or if the injury is not thought serious enough for hospitalization, put him in bed without a pillow under his head. WATCH CLOSELY.
4. Watch closely for bleeding from any of the head cavities and unconsciousness. These are signs that the injury may be quite serious.

FOREIGN BODIES

A listing of the things that small children like to put in their mouths and other body openings would make a book in itself. Do not leave the wick trimmer, nails, sewing needles or any other small objects that a child might conceivably swallow where they are accessible to him.

Treatment for something stuck in the throat or windpipe is given on page 19. It is important to emphasize again that any effect to physically remove anything stuck in the throat may easily become part of the problem rather than its solution. Often, after the initial gagging, hard breathing and coughing, the symptoms will subside. If this happens, get the child in the pickup and to the hospital where x-ray and removal equipment is available.

DISEASE

The common childhood diseases, such as chicken pox, measles and mumps are a fact of life. There are now available immunization shots for many of these hassles and your county medical clinic may offer these shots free. Most of these diseases develop their own immunity in the body once a child has experienced it, and rarely are there any lasting affects or damage if proper medical treatment is available.

There will usually be a warning when any of these diseases are in the community. The word of a new childhood disease outbreak spreads quickly from mother to mother. If your child should begin to have strange outbreaks on his body or experience fever or other symptoms, get him in bed, monitor his temperature frequently and put on a pot of nourishing soup. If the fever gets out of hand wrap the child in cold wet sheets or sponge with cold water. A medical opinion should be sought as these diseases can be very serious.

In dealing with any of the childhood problems, a couple of things to remember are: don't take seriously unsolicited medical advice from your childless friends and neighbors, and summon all the patience you can with the young child who can only cry in an effort to communicate. It is sometimes difficult to determine what is wrong with him. Watch them closely and take temperature often when they are crying without an obvious reason.

EMERGENCY CHILD BIRTH

Not too many generations ago the home was the only proper place for a child to be born, and any written instruction for that function would likely have been found in the Ladies Domestic Science Book somewhere between berry preserves and brine for curing bacon. Home child birth was, for lack of any other place, a necessity and as much a part of homestead life as haying in the early summer. Only after the population began its exodus to the city in quest of the unfulfilled promises of an industrial society did it become fashionable to have children in a hospital. Like their grandmothers did before them, many homestead ladies today are having their children at home. There are some excellent books on the subject of home child birth and if you are considering having your child at home you should study these carefully and have the assistance of a trained midwife or doctor at the time of your delivery.

If the mother should begin labor, though, and the bridge has just been washed out by a storm or the snow is up to the tops of the fence posts on the road, you may find yourselves delivering the baby at home whether or not you had planned it. Once labor begins, the baby will not be inclined to wait until a more convenient time. The information here is presented to help with an EMERGENCY BIRTH.

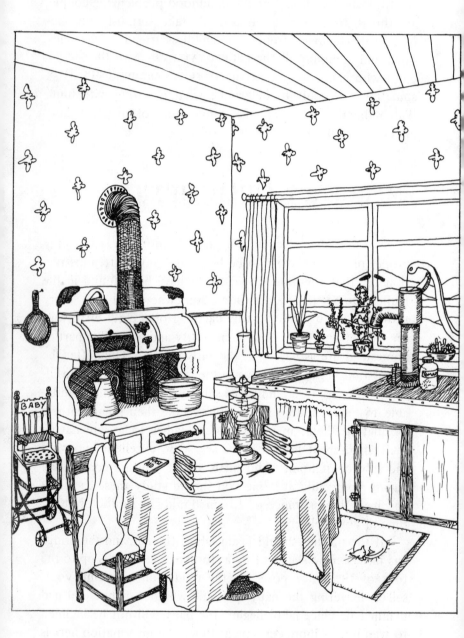

You will need to get together some items in preparation for the delivery.

1. A covered soup pot for sterilization. Fill the pot with soapy water, boil the water for a few minutes, dump and rinse thoroughly, refill it with clean water and bring it to a boil again. This water will be used for sterilization.
2. Lots of clean towels.
3. A clean feed pan or something to receive the afterbirth.
4. A pair of sharp scissors from the sewing kit.
5. Warm clean blankets and clothes for the baby.

Birth of new young is a natural spring happening all around the homestead. As the only animals that have been alienated from the land and natural childbirth for a couple of generations, we need to relearn much of that folk knowledge lost to us during that time. The mother needs to understand that childbirth is a natural thing and that a part of her brain with which she may not even be familiar is equipped by heritage to tell her body the right things to do.

Probably the most important thing in helping a mother with childbirth is to give her reassurance and confidence in herself. She needs to be calm and her muscles relaxed in order for her natural instincts to direct the birth. If she is tense and frightened, it can only prolong the labor and make the delivery difficult and painful.

The beginning of labor is often noted by the discharge of a mass of blood-stained mucus. In other cases, the breaking of the bag of water which the baby is suspended in will soon be followed by labor contractions, although breaking of the water bag may precede labor contractions by several hours. Contractions will become rhythmical and the time between them will become shorter. The mother should be washed well and made comfortable on a clean bed, though if she wants to walk at this time, let her.

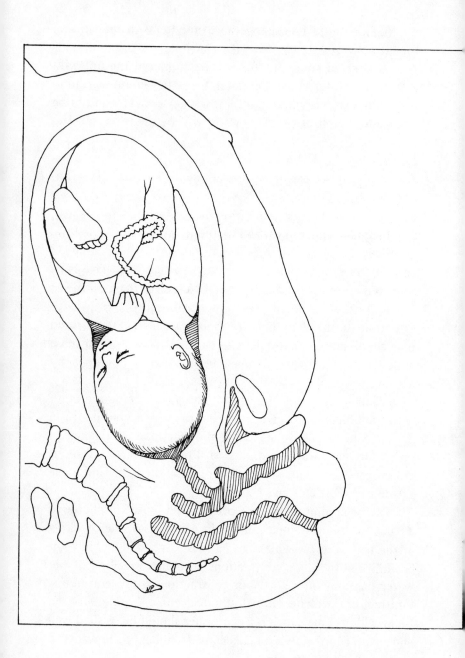

If the baby is going to have to be delivered at home, you should have stoked the fire well for boiling water, and have the delivery room ready by the time the contractions are within five minutes apart. Wash your hands (up to your arms) carefully, at least twice, and rinse in water as hot as you can stand.

By now, she should be in whatever position is most comfortable for her to give birth. Lying on her back is the standard hospital and textbook position, but there are many who feel this is the most difficult position for the mother. Lying on her side, on hands and knees, or squatting, or even standing, are some positions that are more and more frequently being used.

Toward the end of the first stage of labor, the contractions will become stronger and harder, as the opening to the uterus enlarges to let the baby's head enter the birth canal. The mother usually will enter a form of mild shock at this time. She will appear to remove herself from the reality of her experience between contractions.

After the uterus has enlarged, and the baby's head has slipped into the birth canal, the labor pains will ease. The mother will begin to feel a pressure on her rectum as though she were having a hard bowel movement. She may want to help the delivery by bearing down with the final contractions. The first sign of the baby will be the top of his head appearing in the enlarged opening of the vagina. Many times the birth will be completed on the next contraction after the head is born and you must be ready to catch him.

The labor will usually be slow at this time, and you may reassure the mother that the birth is nearly over. If not, you may press gently with your finger on the mother's skin between the anus and the vagina where you will feel the baby's chin. Lift up gently and guide his chin through the opening of the vagina.

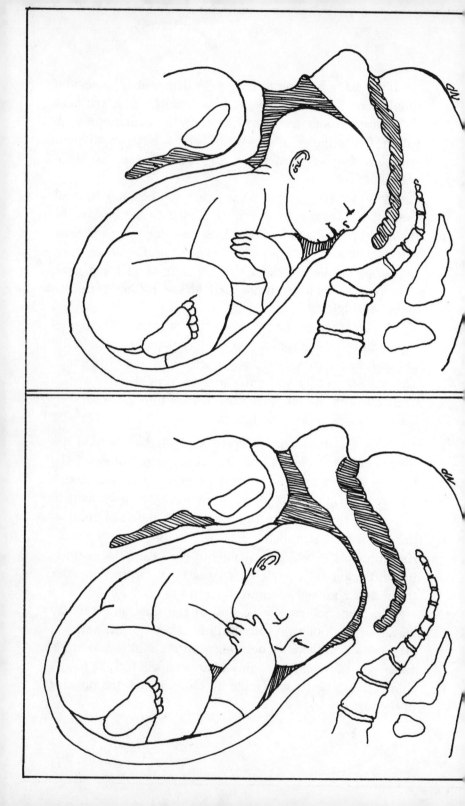

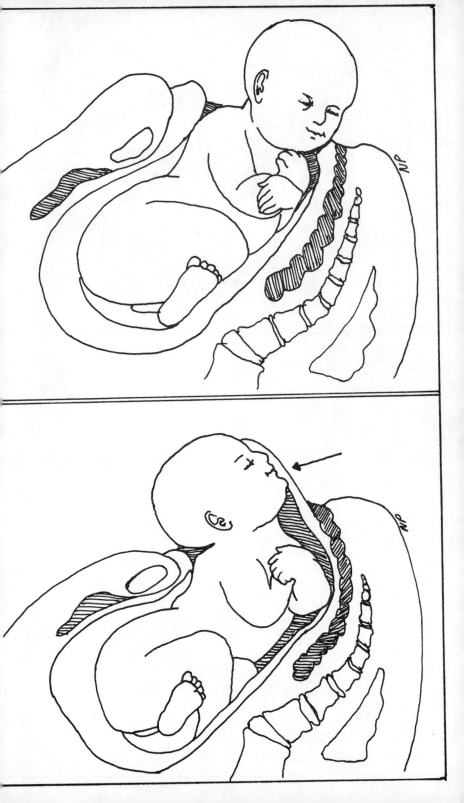

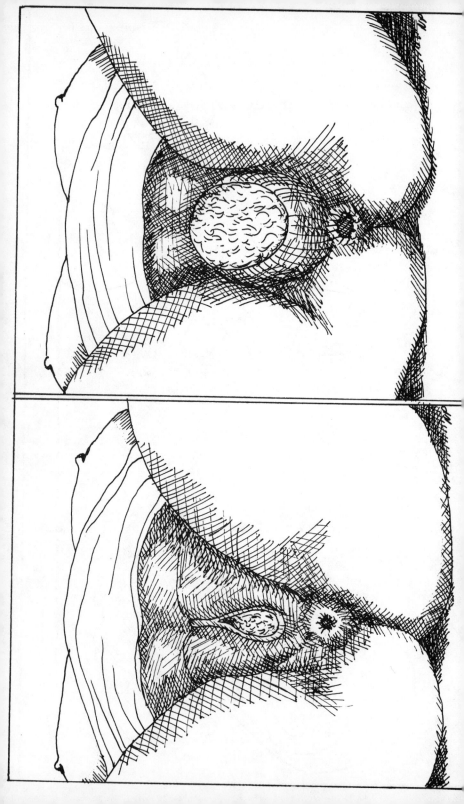

The mother will usually relax after the head has been born. Don't attempt to hurry the birth by pulling on the head of the baby. Permanent injury to the spine and the nerves may result. If the head appears and is still covered by the bag of water, it must be opened so the baby can breathe.

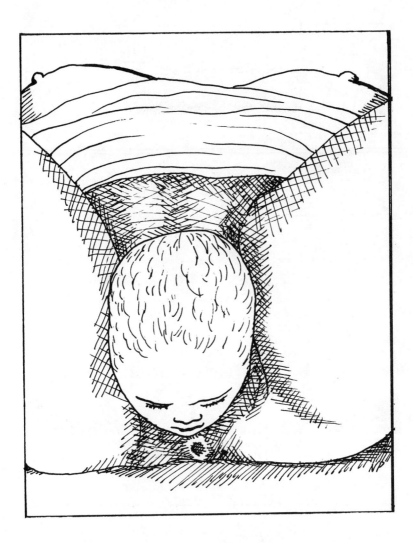

71

Very carefully open it with your fingernails or a sterile knife or scissors. Wipe off the face of the baby with a clean cloth. The mother should be reassured that everything is cool and to bear down on the next contraction. This usually delivers a brand new, slimy blue baby into the world.

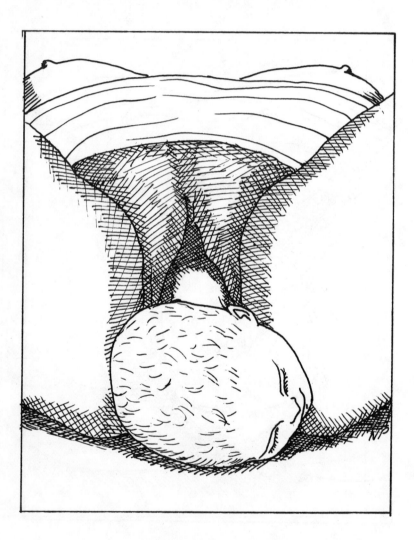

Sometimes the baby's shoulder will be caught on the pelvic bone and some assistance may be needed. If the baby has already started to cry, he may stay in that position as long as he wishes. If he is not crying and breathing, which is usually the case, he must be delivered in the next two contractions as fast as possible, without hurting the mother.

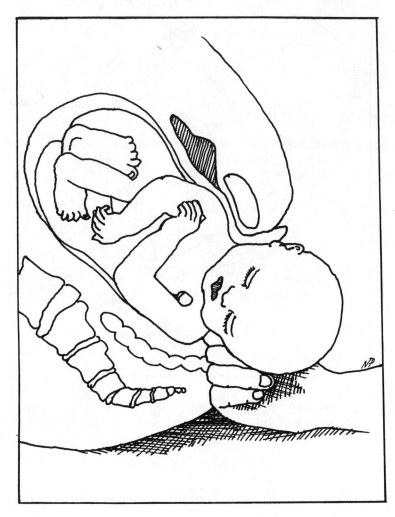

If the shoulders still are not out after two more contractions, locate with your finger the shoulder nearest the mother's backbone. Hook your finger under the arm and pull gently while rotating the shoulder towards the baby's face.

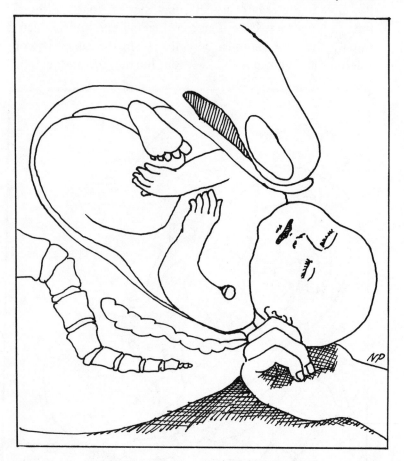

This assistance is normally not required and should only be given when the above methods have not worked. Sometimes the cord is wrapped around the baby's head; wait until the delivery is finished and the baby is completely out before untangling it.

Hold the baby's face down or to the side so he can cough and sneeze the mucus from his mouth and nose. Don't attempt to wash or wipe out his mouth.

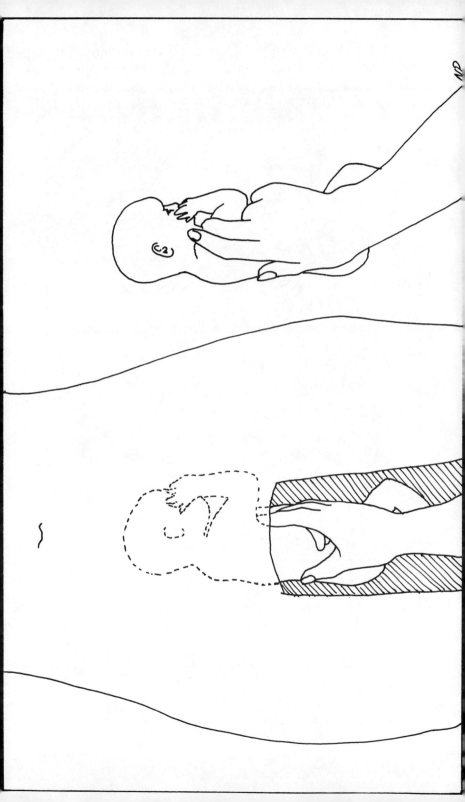

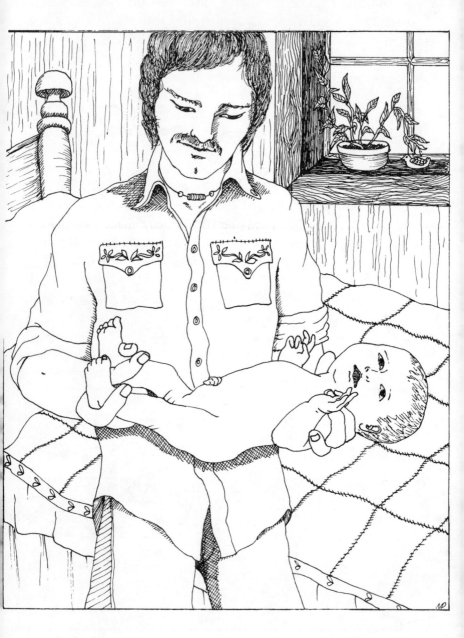

Be sure to hold the slippery little cuss firmly with both your thumb and fingers locked tightly around his ankles as well as a hand under the neck and head. By this time the baby will have started crying and breathing freely. Lay him face down on the mother's abdomen or between her legs, then pat him dry with clean towels, and cover him with warm blankets.

You can now go out on the cabin porch, give three strong rebel yells and have a stiff medicinal belt of whiskey on your way back through the kitchen.

Let the baby cry for a few minutes until the cord has become thinner and changed from bluish color to very pale. About twelve inches from the baby's belly make two tight knots on the end with sterilized cloth tape, about an inch or two apart. These must be tight enough to stop the flow of blood between the baby and the mother. When this is done, cut the cord with the scissors (after they have been sterilized by boiling for at least five minutes).

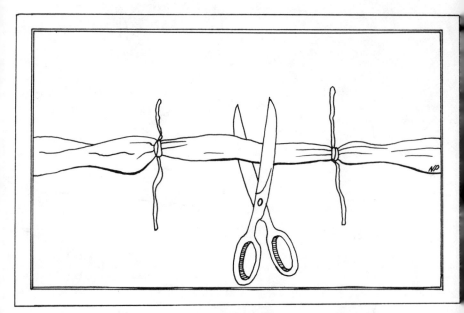

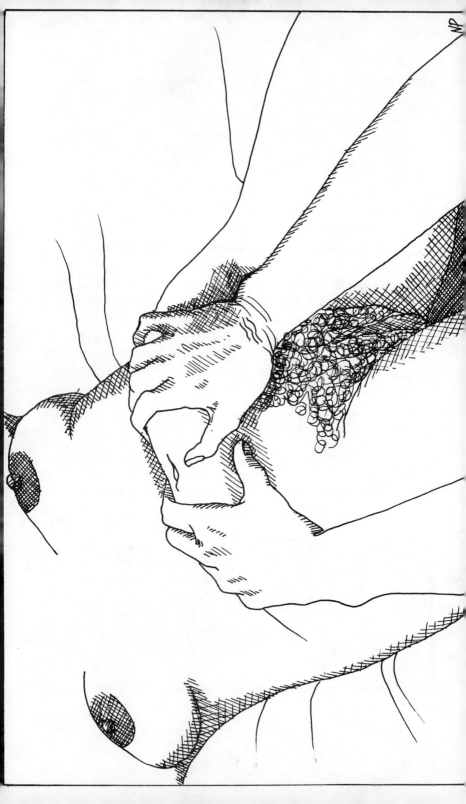

You can now place the baby at the mother's breast; when he starts to suckle, it begins the biological impulse which helps expel the after-birth. The after-birth should be caught in a pan and saved for a doctor or midwife to check that it has been expeled. Don't pull on the after-birth as it may cause hemorraging from the uterus. The after-birth is usually delivered within a few minutes but may sometimes take several hours. If the mother is not bleeding there is no hurry.

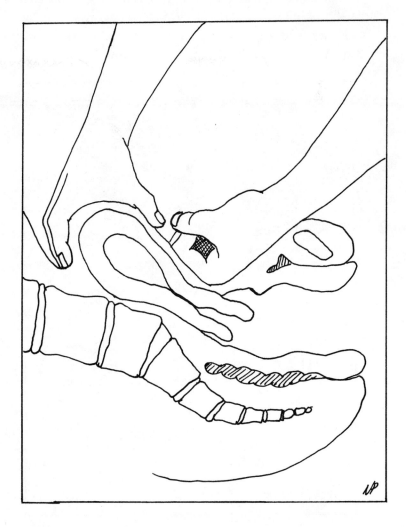

Massage the uterus which will be felt as a soft mass under the now very relaxed stomach muscles. Massage through the stomach by kneading it between your finger tips and base of your hand. As you knead, you will feel it become hard. This is what you want to happen.

With everything under control, you can fix mom a cup of coffee, congratulate her and collapse for a few minutes, to wonder again how it is that nature was designed to work so well.

When the mother feels like it, clean her off and change the sheets on the bed. Don't clean the baby by wiping, as he comes into the world with a special finish on his skin for protection. Pat him gently with a clean soft towel.

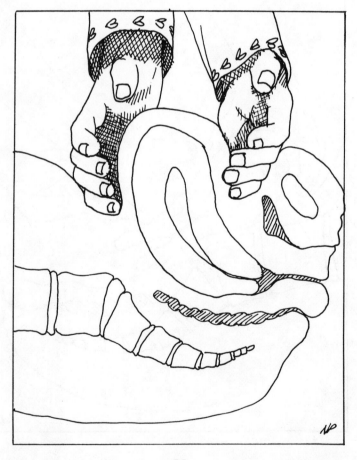

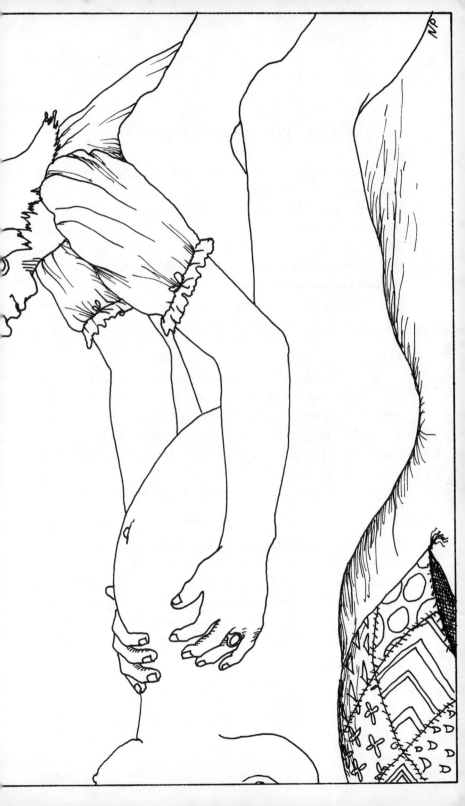

UNUSUAL DELIVERIES

Most deliveries will be normal as above; and delivery could easily be assisted by an intelligent ten year old. Sometimes the baby will be uncooperative and will come out face up or even butt or feet first. A face up delivery is treated as a normal delivery, and in a couple of days the face will lose that "born through the washing machine wringer" appearance and be normal.

Although unusual, a breech birth, when the baby is backing out, is still common enough to take into consideration. In a breech delivery the mother should be in a hands and knees position.

When the baby being born has progressed as far as his naval in a breech birth, the head must be delivered within the next eight to ten minutes. Normally the mother's efforts will accomplish this. If after five or six minutes the baby is not born, you may pull gently on the baby's legs, but never before the naval is out. Do not let the baby's back turn towards the mother's back; it should be sideways or facing the mother's stomach.

The arms of the baby should be brought out before the head if the arms do not appear first. When the armpit appears, gently press the shoulder toward the spine. This will usually free the arm. If not, insert two fingers into the vagina nearest the back bone and manipulate the arm across the baby's chest and out. Then repeat with the other arm. If necessary, the baby may be rotated gently to accomplish this.

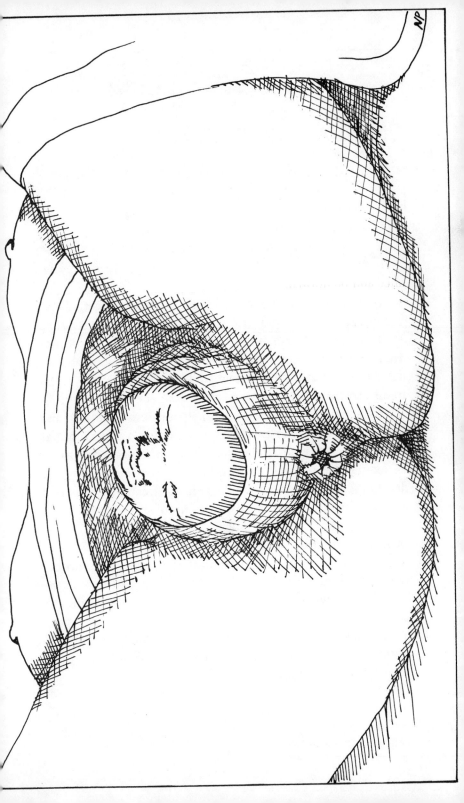

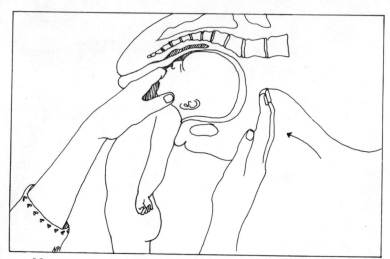

Next, reach in and carefully insert your finger in the baby's mouth. Press his chin onto his chest. Avoid possible spinal damage by not pulling on the baby. If he is still not delivered, use as much pressure as you can, without hurting him, on the mother's abdomen while holding the baby's chin to his chest.

This would be an exceptionally difficult delivery and these methods should be used only after you are certain that they are necessary. If the head still can't be delivered, make an air passage so the baby can breathe (see Illus.) and get a doctor. As long as the baby is able to breathe he can wait indefinitely. Do not try to force the birth by using brute strength; the result may be death or permanent injury to the mother or the child.

If a hand should appear first at the vagina, the mother must be hospitalized. This means the baby is crosswise in the birth canal and surgery will be required to complete the birth.

A heavy but short flow of blood out of the mother is normal but excessive bleeding after giving birth is fairly unusual. If massaging the uterus as described earlier doesn't stop the flow, you may try using the two pressure methods on the uterus as illustrated. At this point it is obvious you are going to need help. If you are using enough pressure to cause pain after delivery, it is too much.

SNAKE BITE

It seems that lots of the cheap land available to homesteaders is cheap because it is steep or hilly, covered with rock and brush, and inhabitable only by lower life critters.

Some of these are poisonous. Probably the most dangerous is the snake.

I remember that Grandpa Wilson, back on the old homestead, lived in constant fear of snakebite. His defense for snakebite was to keep a pint of local moonshine at important points around the barnyard. This way, if he was to get a notion that he might be bitten while feeding the hogs, he would stop by the shed and have a good snort. Similarly, bottles lay in wait in the stables, under the eaves of the chicken coop, and one in a hollow of the oak tree in the middle of the barnyard.

Of course Grandma must not have had any faith in this method, because Grandpa always said that she wasn't to know about his fears on account of he didn't want to "worry her none". She said, though, that her two big calico cats did a fine job of keeping snakes away from the yard, which may have been a more sensible plan.

There are four species of poisonous snakes in the continental U.S. Their descriptions and characteristics are beyond the scope of this effort, but you should determine which snakes might be common in your own area. Until then, complete respect should be shown for any snake. Don't kill all snakes though. The non-poisonous ones are very good helpers in controlling populations of pests in the garden and the feed shed.

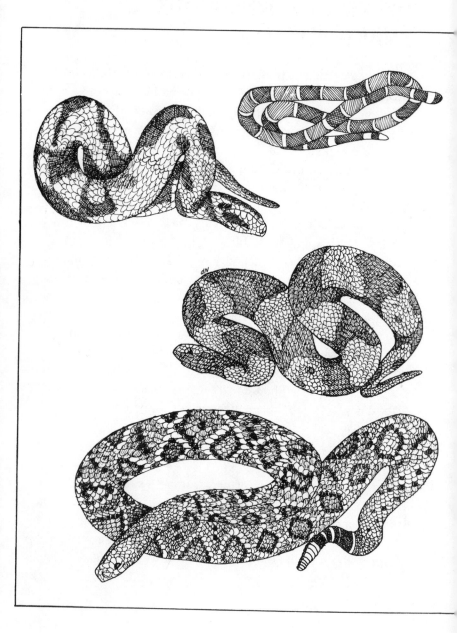

TREATING A POISONOUS
SNAKE BITE

Anyone bitten by a snake should get medical attention as soon as possible. If you're out in the back forty, though, and the pick-up is in town for groceries, there are some things you can do.

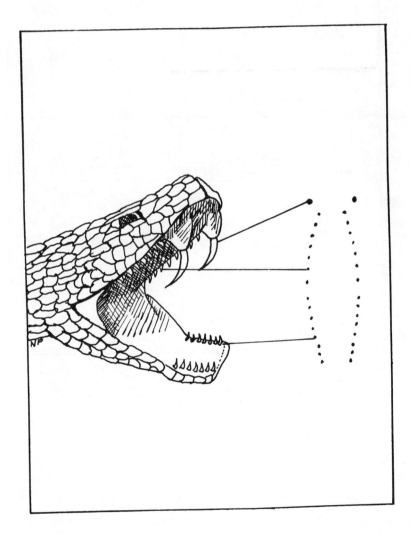

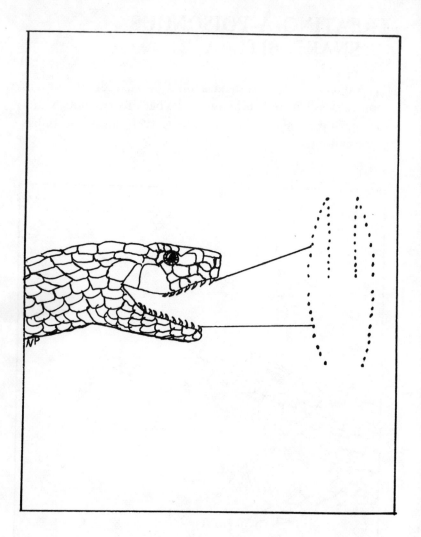

Snake bite is rarely lethal if good immediate first-aid and medical treatment is used.

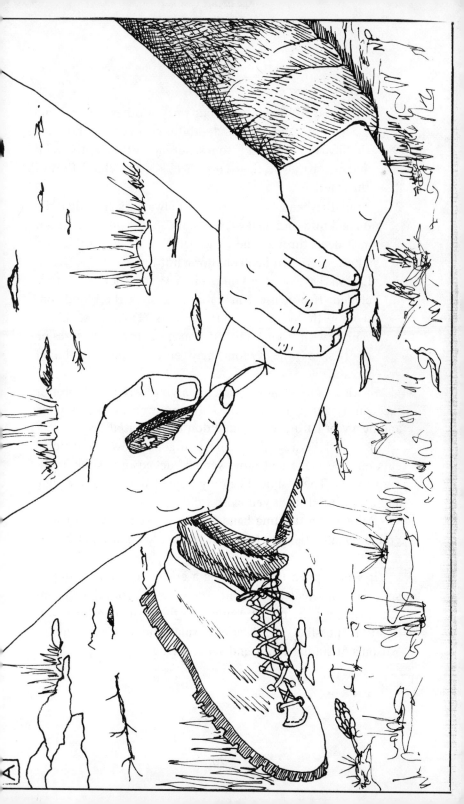

1. First tear off a piece of your shirt or other material and tie a snug band around the bite, between the bite and the heart. The band is to restrict blood flow in the veins and must not be tight enough to restrict blood flow in the arteries.

2. After the band is tied, use your always clean and sterile Buck knife and make cross cuts about a quarter of an inch deep through the fang marks. If at all possible, use a knife sterilized in alcohol or a hot flame.

3. If you have a snake bite kit, use the suction cup included. If not, use your mouth to suck the blood containing the venom from the cuts. Do not suck the venom with your mouth if you have any open sores or cavities, as the venom may enter your own blood stream.

By this time we hope you are on your way to a doctor or the county nurse in your area. In any event, avoid running and heavy or hard exercise, and don't get excited.

If it will be a while before you get to town, additional cuts may be made and more venom sucked out as the swelling spreads. There should be only a small amount of bleeding and a flow of clear or yellowish fluid.

Raise the restricting band if swelling goes beyond where you originally tied it. It is best to tie a second band before removing the first.

If you happen to be hunting a critter for Sunday dinner and have a medical student friend with you, you might administer a shot of anti-venom on the spot. If not, stay as quiet as possible, *don't* use a small amount of Grandpa Wilson's or similar tonic, and get to a Doc.

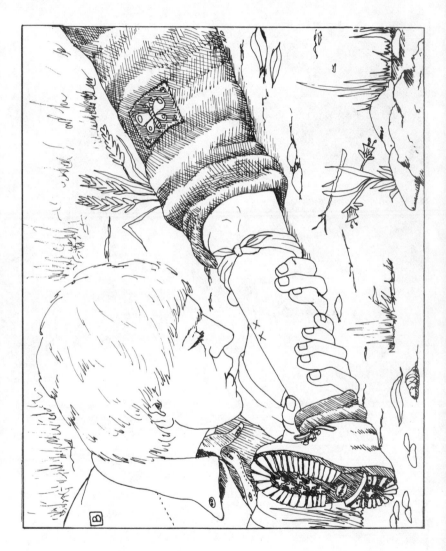

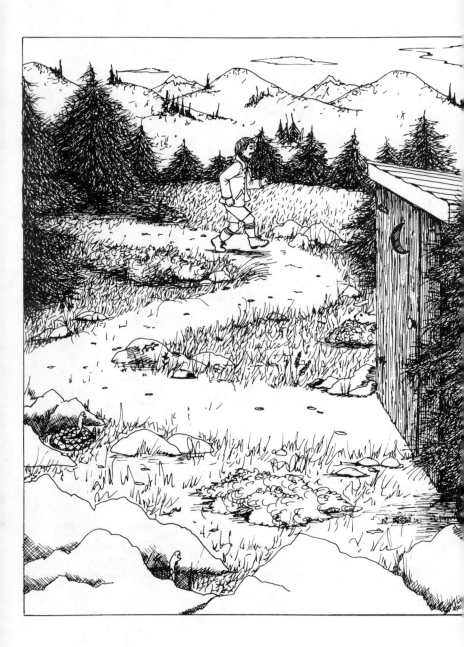

The kids should be especially warned about snakes and what to do as soon as they are old enough to relate to them. Kids seem to like to play in the same places as snakes are found, and are naturally inquisitive about the other critters that inhabit the common biological community.

The same first-aid as for people may be used for the goats, your dog or whatever. Animals in good health normally will recover well after a period of being sick.

Shortly after her first snake rap, four-year-old Lisa ran excitedly into the kitchen one warm spring afternoon to edify all with the knowledge that a snake had taken over the tool shed. To the first contingent to arrive she proudly pointed at a very large angle worm crawling on the dirt in a corner. At least she was aware.

THE BEES AND THE PEOPLE

I sure do love those critters while they are making honey in their hives under the apple trees, but they can be downright ornery when you are picking in the blackberry patch. Their cousins, the wasps and hornets, are even more formidable. They can easily defend the dead oak in the pasture from my chain saw. These of God's creatures have the ability to remove their stingers and do it again; thus a colony of them can make life uncomfortable. Honey bees are good for only one sting, and they give their lives in this heroic effort, leaving their stinger imbedded in the victim, where it continues for some time to inject poison. Bee venom is said to be as potent, gram for gram, as rattlesnake venom, though bees don't inject as much as a snake due to their smaller size.

TREATMENT

1.   Remove the stinger by scraping with the edge of a pocket knife or something else sharp. Don't squeeze it with anything, as this will force out more venom.
2.   Make a paste of baking soda and water and apply this to the sting, or soak the sting in Epsom salts for relief.

Some people who have been stung many times by bees are extremely sensitive to bee sting. They are subject to anaphylactic shock, characterized by difficult breathing, restlessness, spotted skin, headache and cough, or the appearance of being in traumatic shock. If someone is aware they react this way to a sting, a doctor can provide an emergency kit of ephinephrine (a heart stimulant) to inject after a bee sting, which will relieve the symptoms. This kit should be nearby at all times.

Immediate medical help is required if the above is not available. Sometimes hay fever or cold capsules will help the victim. Any antihistamine is likely to help.

Remember, the bee sting can be fatal to some people. Never treat a sting lightly, and especially watch children for a severe reaction to sting.

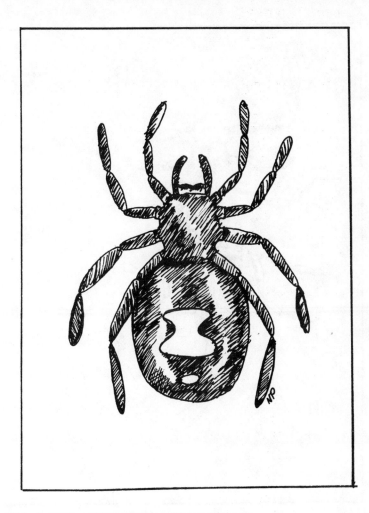

BLACK WIDOW SPIDERS

Old wood buildings and dark cool places are popular with black widow spiders. This makes them feel quite at home on the homestead. The black widow is easily distinguished by a red spot on its belly. Especially watch for signs of this disagreeable critter in the outhouse. She can turn an otherwise enjoyable and contemplative morning reading period into a very painful experience.

The symptoms of black widow bite are severe stomach pain, swelling, dilation of pupils, partial collapse and sometimes convulsions.

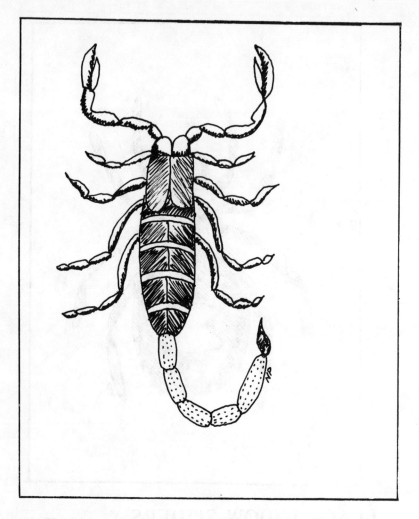

Use the same first-aid treatment as for snake bites. In addition a plaster of baking soda may also be applied.

Most emergency medical facilities will have anti-venoms available. A black widow bite is rarely fatal if treated properly. Do not get excited or in any way stimulate the heart.

The bite of the tarantula is very similar to the black widow bite and may be treated the same.

Scorpion stings are more serious and affect the nervous system. If your homestead is in an area that has scorpions, you should consult your county medical facility or a doctor about keeping a supply of anti-venom on hand.

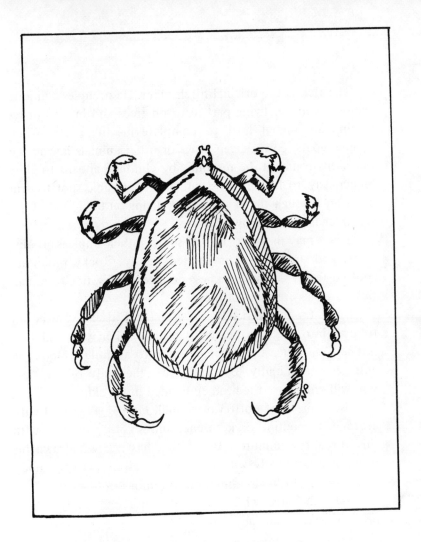

TICK BITE

The tick is not poisonous but rates very high on the list of homestead pests. There is no practical way to convince this nasty little critter that he is not welcome on his human neighbors and their domestic animals.

The tick is the original hitch hiker. He occupies a unique ecological niche, living part in or on trees and brush but requiring an animal host to complete his life cycle. When people, goats, cows, sheep, dogs or other animals invade the tick's environment, he responds by climbing aboard to cling tenaciously to his new host and seek a suitable spot to drill his head through the skin, to begin living on the blood of the victim chance has thrown his way.

Ticks may be carriers for some rather unpleasant diseases, and are not to be treated lightly. Rocky mountain spotted fever, sleeping sickness or encephalitis, tick fever and tick paralysis are some of these.

Don't try to physically pull a tick off after he has begun to drill into the skin, which is usually when you will first notice him. Once the tick has begun to assimilate blood, he enlarges very rapidly. By pulling off the body of the tick, you will only leave the head embedded in the skin.

Use a piece of cotton or a small cloth soaked well with acetone, turpentine or kerosene, and smother the tick with this for a few minutes. If the tick has not withdrawn his head, as he generally will, you may carefully twist the body in a counter clock-wise direction to remove it.

Wash the area with soap and water and apply a light paste of baking soda and water.

Do not use tweezers to try and dig a tick out, or try to burn it out with a lit cigarette as in the old John Wayne flicks. If a tick head should be broken off and left in the skin, it should be removed surgically by a doctor.

SHOCK

Shock follows or accompanies stress to the body and is present to one degree or another in nearly all accidents, burns or other injuries. Since science doesn't fully understand shock yet, it is obviously beyond this book to give a definitive analysis of it here. It is only important to know that if someone has fallen out of the apple-tree on his head, and is walking around doing weird things, he needs to be treated for shock.

Shock is a general slow down of vital body functions and is a natural biological defense the body has. In severe cases it can be fatal. It is important, then, to be able to recognize and treat shock right after other obvious treatment such as for bleeding or not breathing has been accomplished.

SYMPTOMS OF SHOCK

1. Pale or ashen skin.
2. Skin cold and damp.
3. Low body temperature.
4. Shallow breathing.
5. Rapid and weak pulse.
6. Psychological Anesthesia, which is the long way to say freaking out and doing strange things like trying to drive home after wrecking the truck and breaking an arm or bashing your head on the dash.

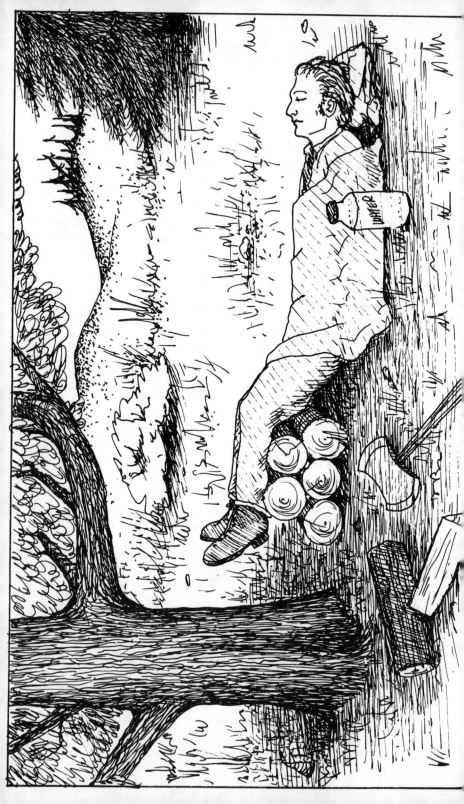

TREATMENT FOR SHOCK

1. Get the victim into a reclining position, with his feet higher than his head.
2. Keep him warm with blankets, feed sacks or whatever you've got handy. Put them under as well as over the victim.
3. Give the victim as much fluid as he/she will take. With most homesteaders, just set a case of cold beer beside them and they will soon have replaced the precious lost body fluids.

A note about alcohol may be in order. Alcohol in the blood seems to promote bleeding and should not be given to anyone with serious bleeding or possible internal hemorrhage. Plain old spring water or teas are a lot safer by far.

ELECTRICAL SHOCK

Of course all good homesteaders adhere carefully to the uniform building code and the latest approved practices when wiring the cabin and barns, so electrical shock should never be a problem. If you should be struck by a sudden bolt of lightning while milking the goat or the storm knocks over the power lines while you are trying to get all of the animals in the barn, it would be healthy and just good sense to have an idea of what to do.

Electrical shock may cause unconsciousness, paralyze breathing, stop the heart completely or cause it to twitch ineffectively, cause burns and otherwise cause general all-around discomfort.

Get the victim separated from the electrical current immediately. Be careful not to also become a victim yourself. If possible cut the current at the main switch or breaker. Otherwise, use something non-conductive such as a stick or rope to separate the victim and the source. Do not touch a person who is still exposed to the current.

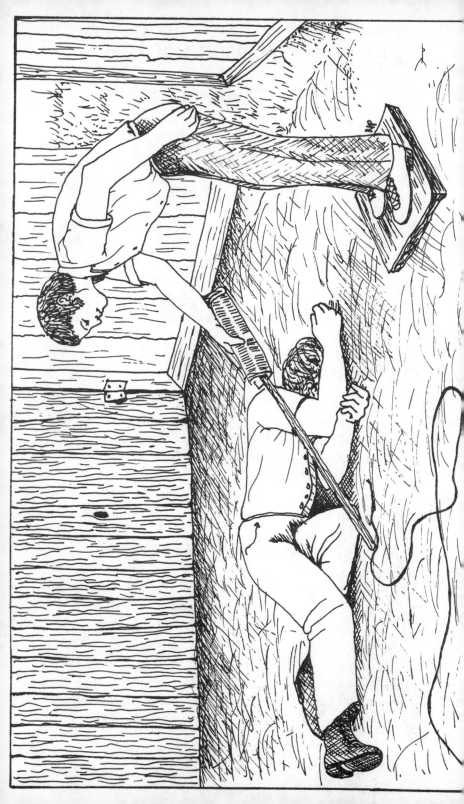

Begin mouth to mouth breathing, external heart massage if required and treat for traumatic shock as above.

The seriousness of shock should not be underestimated but prompt recognition and treatment of the symptoms will most always prevent more serious results.

Since even 110 volt house current can be fatal, it is important that wiring and appliances are safe and grounded, especially in the kitchen, bathroom and milk barn, where water is common. Water seems to aid the human body in becoming an excellent electrical conductor.

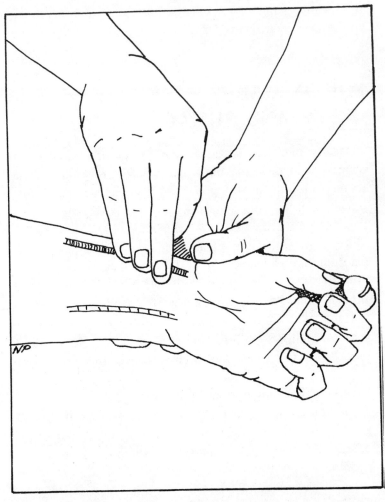

HOW TO FEEL AND MEASURE PULSE

Pulse and the pulse rate are vital life signs giving important clues about the victim's condition. The pulse is the heart beat forcing blood into the arteries in the body. It can be felt and measured anywhere on the body where an artery is close to the skin. The easiest place is the underside of the wrist and can be felt and measured by holding your finger tips firmly against it. A normal pulse rate is between sixty and seventy heart beats per minute.

POISON OAK, IVY AND SUMAC

Many new homesteaders make their first agonizing encounter with these insidious plants before they have learned to recognize them during *all* the different seasons. Here in our own parts, poison oak is rampant, largely due to poor logging and grazing practices, which create ideal growing conditions. In fact, if there was some commercial value for the plant, homesteaders could at least probably pay off their mortgage on the place in no time at all. We have found, though, that "the girls" (our goats) happily convert some poison oak into very good milk (which is said to pass on some immunity to humans who drink it). It would be foolish, though, to attempt a large scale eradication program with goats, because tethering them in the poison oak patch for a long time may poison a good goat.

If you are just moving onto your homestead, it would be good to find someone to carefully show you as many stages of development of the particular plant in your area as possible.

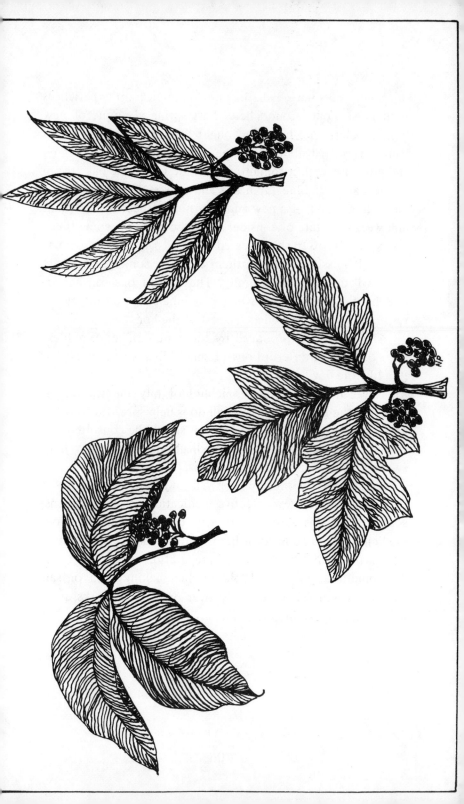

Some folks have had some mighty unpleasant experiences with poison oak around here. Last spring a couple of new homesteaders who had just bought the forty across the road were so excited about their new land that they celebrated the purchase with a romantic interlude under the oak tree in a fine patch of blue lupines — and poison oak. A couple of days later they had a new and profound respect for the plant and were in a state of considerable discomfort for some time.

Never burn freshly cleared poison oak, ivy, or sumac plants. If possible just pile them carefully some place where they will deteriorate naturally. The irritant oils can be carried by the smoke, and when it is inhaled it can infect the respiratory tract, as well as the rest of the body.

The symptoms produced by these are patches of reddening skin with later eruptions of small blisters and sores that itch like the devil.

Never use any type of alcohol or oily medication on these, as the only thing they will do is help spread it to other areas. In really severe cases, a doctor should be consulted, for there are some prescription medications that will relieve swelling and other allergic symptoms.

Treatment for most poison oak, ivy, and sumac cases is limited to a very few effective medications, usually lotions, soaps or creams designed to dry up the infection. Folk medicines made from local herbs and plants may be as much help as many of the commercial preparations.

Sometimes just good old kitchen baking soda or salt moistened and spread liberally over open sores works quite well to dry up the infection and stop the itching.

STRAINS AND SPRAINS

In other life styles muscle strains and sprains of skeletal joints are considered an accident. The homesteader usually learns quickly that these problems are common to the more unusual activities of putting a farm together. Technically, a strained muscle is one that has been partly torn by a hard, unexpected pull on the muscle.

The most common muscle strain around the homestead is usually the lower back. Don't leave yourself open for these kinds of injuries. You only get one back to last a whole lifetime. When it comes time to hoist the thirty foot log that you have hewn into a timber for the cabin, get out your banjos and fiddles, a bottle of red wine, some home fried chicken, and some salad. Then invite a few neighbors over for a "timber raisin'." With enough help to do the job, no one will get hurt and afterwards you can enjoy an afternoon of good food and maybe even some fiddlin' and pickin'.

Anyone who experiences a strained muscle will know it when they feel the sharp, tearing pain. In the case of a back strain, the pain may go all the way down into the legs. Sometimes there will be muscle spasms with very sharp pain. Stiffness and pain on movement are later signs, and in the case of a minor strain, may be the first noticeable sign if the strain wasn't felt at the time it happened.

Rest the strained muscles in the most comfortable position you can, using pillows or whatever. Hot wet towels or other heat on the muscle and gentle massage near the strain will also help.

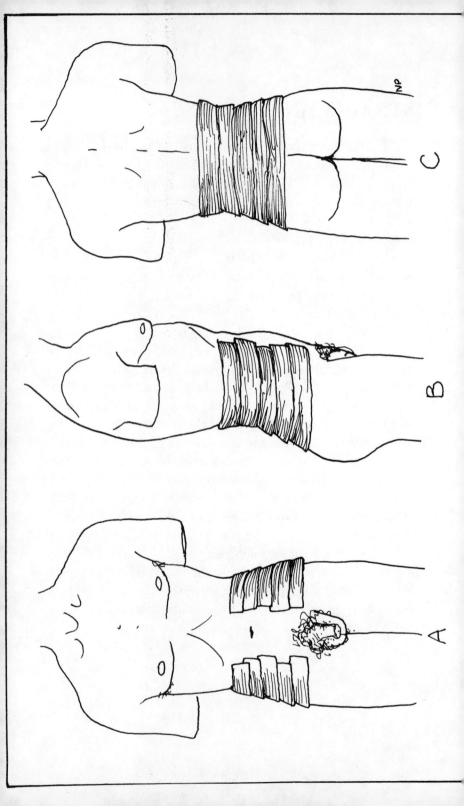

A   B   C

One of the neighbors, an old timer who lives on the ridge, swears by this cure for back ache. He digs some cowslip roots, brews them in a soup pot for an hour on the woodstove, and pours this into a hot bath. While soaking in the bath he drinks two cups of hot brandy and water. Don't rightly know if this works but at least the brandy may make you not care about the backache.

Many times a strained muscle will benefit from being wrapped. This will limit movement and compression on the muscle. A method of using three inch wide adhesive tape to support a strained back muscle is shown in the illustration. This is a good temporary support, but any back strain severe enough to require support should be checked by a doctor.

CHARLEY HORSE

Everyone has had the old "charley horse" at one time. This is a tightening of a muscle into a seeming knot from over exertion of the muscle. Treatment is the same as for a strained muscle except the muscle should be kneaded, massaged, and a conscious effort should be made to relax. As soon as it subsides, rest and avoid using the muscle until it is comfortable again. A charley horse will mostly occur in the calf muscle of the leg or the bicep in the upper arm.

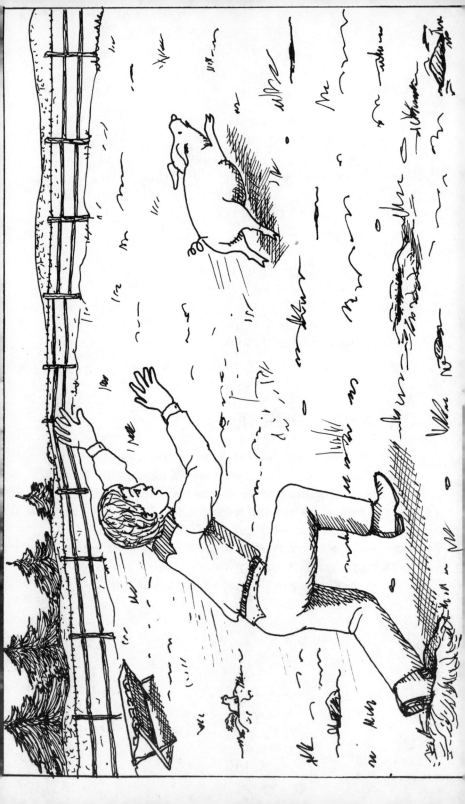

SPRAINS

A sprain is what you are likely to get when you are trying to catch the weaner pigs in the pasture, and just about the time you are ready to dive for one, you get your foot caught in a squirrel hole. The first symptoms of a sprain, then, are often a series of incoherent four letter epithets from the victim, followed by sharp pain, rapid swelling and nasty discoloration.

Sometimes it is hard to tell without x-ray whether or not it is, in fact, a sprain or a fracture. A sprain may be from quite minor to very severe with actual slipping of the bone in the affected joint. Medically, a sprain is damage to the ligaments and cartilage (those things that keep the bones together in a workable fashion). They result from twisting or wrenching a joint in a direction in which it was not designed to be moved.

TREATMENT

First aid treatment for strains and sprains is to elevate and rest the sprained joint or muscle, and apply ice packs or whatever cold application is available for the first 24 hours. Wrap the injury firmly with an elastic bandage, support and immobilize it with a sling if it is possible. Don't use adhesive in place of an elastic bandage because it will not expand if swelling increases. An elastic bandage is easily removed and re-wrapped if it becomes too tight.

After the first 24 hours, apply hot wet towels or soak the joint or muscle in water as hot as possible and massage it gently with your fingers. This will aid in re-absorbing the blood around the injured joint which is the cause of swelling.

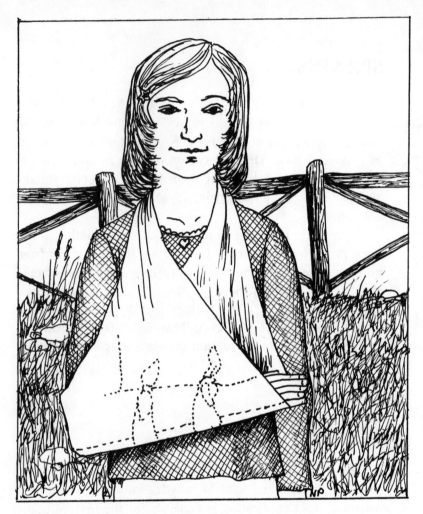

When the swelling has started to go down, and if it is absolutely necessary for the injured to use the joint, you may wrap it more firmly with adhesive tape. This normally should only be done under medical direction. If, with use of the limb, swelling should begin again, remove the tape and use the elastic bandage.

If a fracture is suspected, of course the joint should be splinted and the victim taken to a medical facility for treatment. Not infrequently, a severe sprain may also involve chipping of bone in the joint which, if left untreated, may cause later complications.

BROKEN BONES

Yes, human bones are fragile and homestead life can be hard on them. There are two medical classes of broken bones. The simple fracture is just a broken bone. The compound fracture is a broken bone that also breaks through the skin, making the whole thing uglier. A fracture is easily recognized. Folks who break a bone often hear the distinct snap and feel the grating. If you are not sure Johnny broke his arm when he fell out of the tree house, don't ask him to move it to see if it is broken. Besides loss of the use of a limb, look for deformity, swelling and discoloration. In a compound fracture the broken bone may protrude.

If Aunt Maude is up from the city and breaks a leg tripping over an exposed tree root on her way to the outhouse in the middle of the night, you will have to get into action. Don't move anyone with a break, or even a suspected break, unnecessarily. It is best not to move him at all, but it is hard to get a doctor out at night to fix Aunt Maude's broken leg beside the outhouse.

Any broken bone must be immobilized before moving the victim. A splint may be fashioned from nearly anything rigid. The broken pitchfork handle, boards, sticks, even a thick newspaper can be used to set a fracture. The splint must be applied so it not only holds each end of the break but also immobilizes the joint above and below the break. The splint may be tied with nearly anything convenient, strips of torn cloth, rope, baling wire, suspenders, etc.

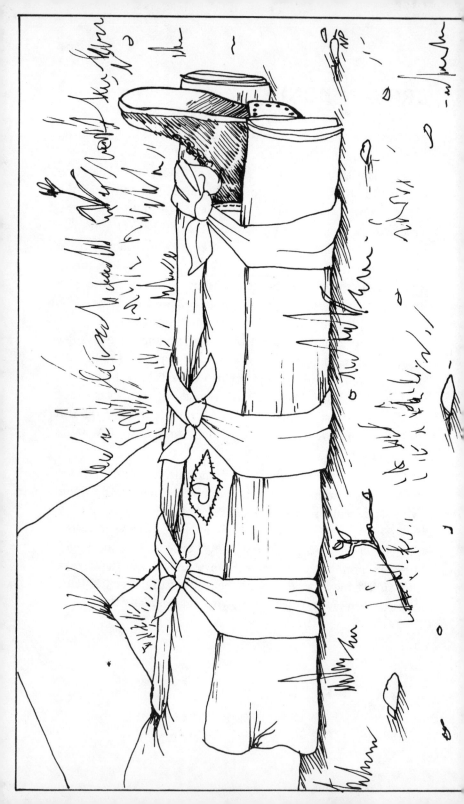

Always treat even a suspected break as if it really was. If the break is compound, cover the wound with sterile gauze or clean cloth and control the bleeding. Never attempt to push a protruding bone back in place. After bleeding is stopped, splint the limb as above. Treat victim for shock. If unconsciousness occurs from the pain, be ready to give mouth-to-mouth breathing. Using a stretcher, a blanket, a plank or whatever, get the victim into a vehicle and to a Doc.

TREATMENT FOR
SPECIFIC BREAKS

Again, the important thing for any break is to prevent the broken bone ends from moving and treat for shock.

LEG

With padding of some kind in place, tie board splinters on each side of the leg. The inside board should go from the groin to past the heel. The outside board should go from the hip to past the heel. If you don't happen to have two pieces of kiln dried 1 x 4 white oak of the right length, or even a couple of dead branches from a tree, you may place jackets, blankets, etc., between the victim's legs and tie the two legs together.

FOOT OR TOES

Remove or cut away the victim's shoe and sock. If winter is coming and they are new boots, by all means try not to cut the boot off. This may help prevent victim from later experiencing extreme frost bite. Bandage the foot well over a padded dressing or a small pillow.

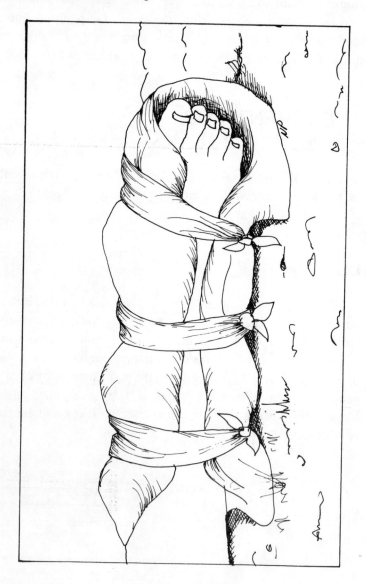

KNEE CAP

Tie a splint to the bottom of the leg, from heel to buttock.

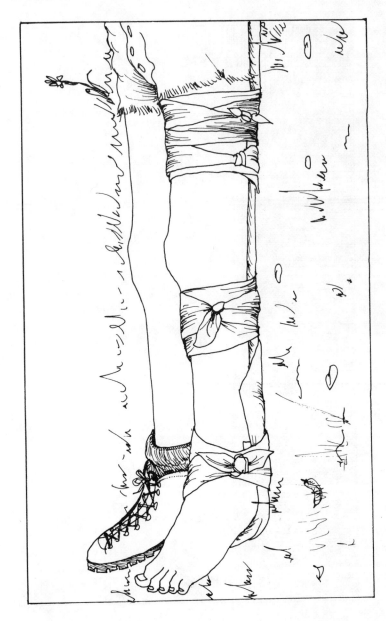

THIGH

Use a wide board splint from the shoulder to the foot.
Tie legs together with padding between them.

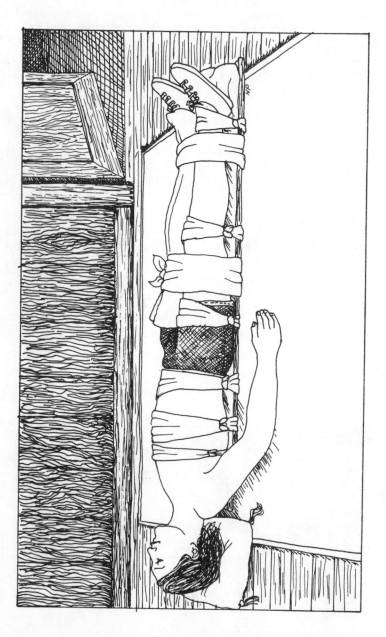

ELBOW

Splint a broken elbow the way it is, do not move it. This will require some creative thinking, but the idea is to splint as much of the arm as possible.

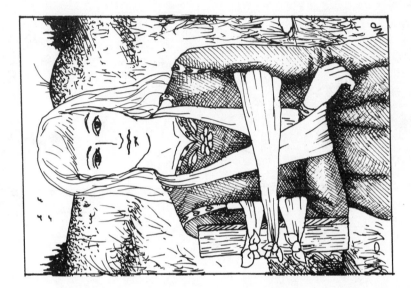

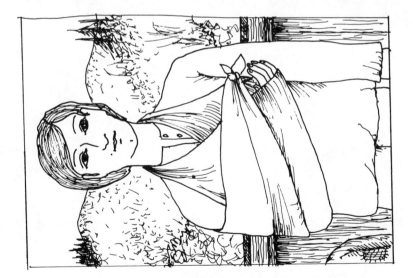

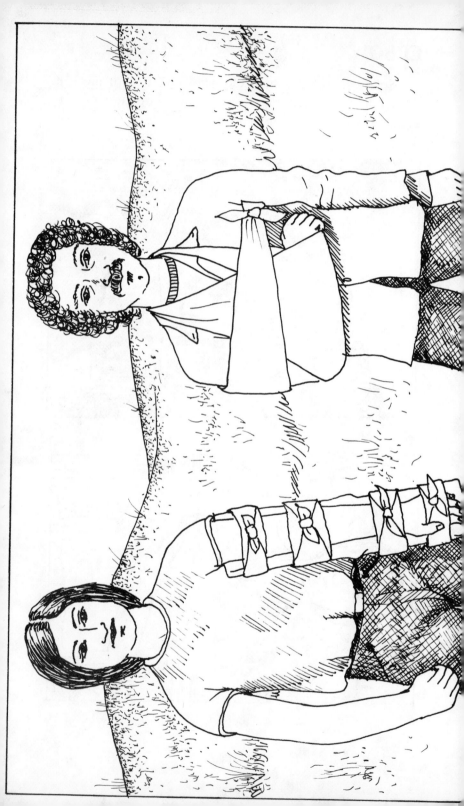

FOREARM OR WRIST

Tie splints from the elbow to the fingers on the top and the bottom. Support the forearm in a sling with the hand higher than the elbow.

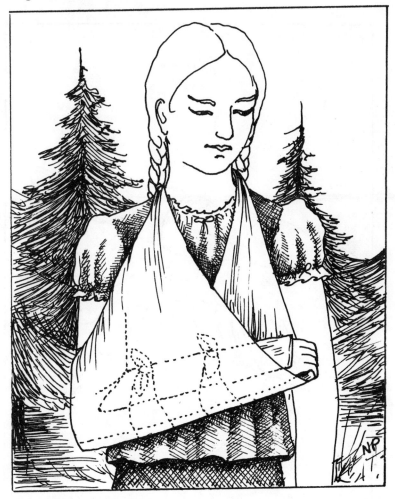

HAND

Use a splint on the front of the hand from the finger tips to the middle of the forearm. Support in a sling.

FINGER

Apply splint to the front of the finger.

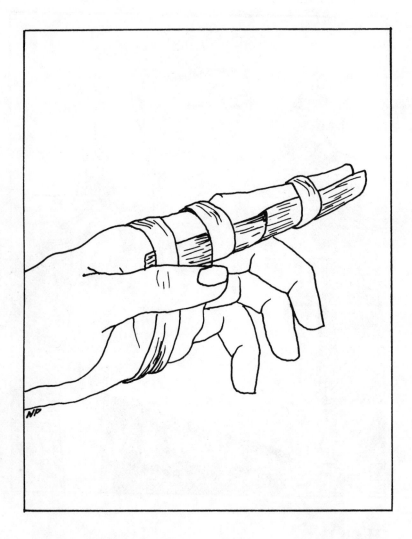

COLLARBONE

Put padding between the arm and the chest, support the arm in a sling and tie the arm to the side of the body.

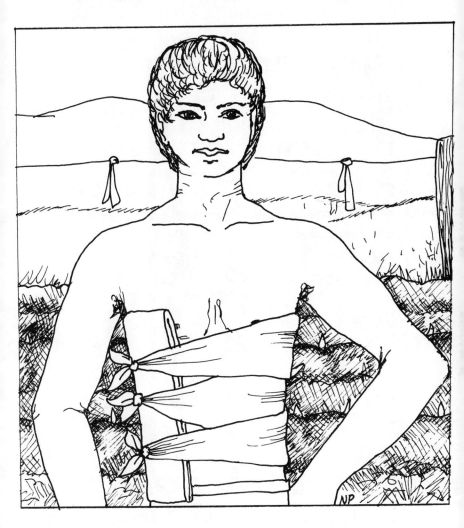

RIBS

Tie bandages loosely over the broken rib with the knots on the opposite side of the break. If the ribs are caved in or the victim is coughing blood, do not attempt to bandage. Treat for shock, or breathing if necessary while getting victim to medical help.

PELVIS

Using a sheet or a blanket wrap the victim from just below the chest past the hips. Tie the legs together with padding between and transport the victim secured to a rigid support.

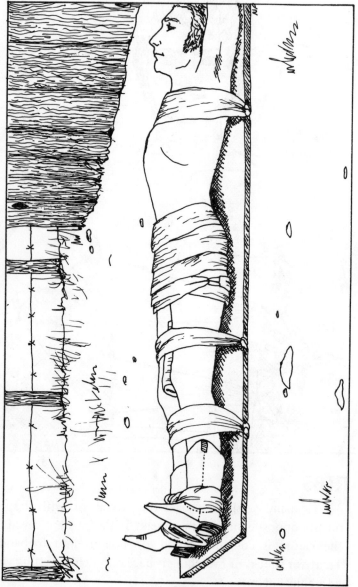

BACK AND NECK

Back and neck fractures are very dangerous. Death or permanent paralysis can easily result. If a victim of an accident has any pain in those areas, treat them as a fracture. Do not attempt to move the victim in any way. Cover the victim and get help.

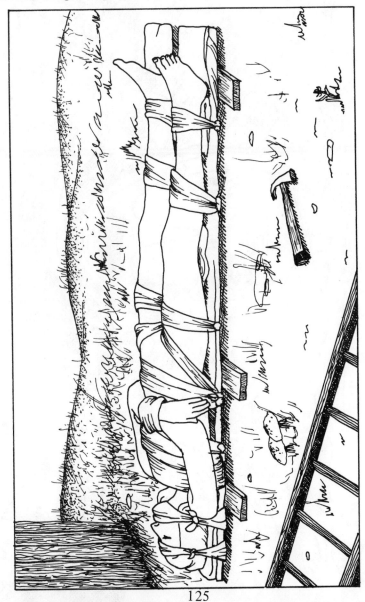

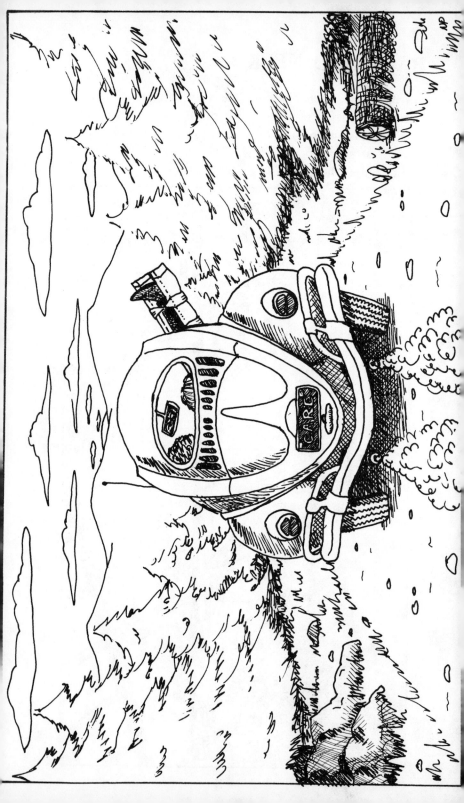

HEAD

Lay a concussion victim on his back with the head slightly raised. Watch his breathing closely. If the victim is choking on blood or vomiting, lower the head and turn it to one side so the mouth will drain. Cover the wound with sterile gauze and tie loosely with cloth strips. Treat the victim for shock but do not give him any stimulants. Transport the victim to help immediately. Brain surgery is generally beyond the scope of most homestead first aiders.

TRANSPORTATION

Transporting the severely injured homesteader is often a necessity. Don't, unless more serious injury may occur or death may result. This purposely leaves a lot unsaid. You will have to make the decisions at the time based on circumstances that have possibly never before been recorded in the annals of modern medicine. There must be an education of complicating the injuries by moving the victim against losing valuable time. Unlike the folks back in the city who merely have to pick up the phone to summon a corps of ambulances, fire trucks, rescue teams and the clergyman of their choice, you will need to apply some creative thinking and do some heavy decision making. We will try to give you some basics.

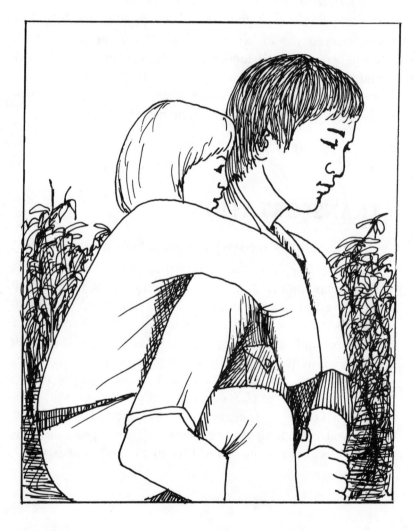

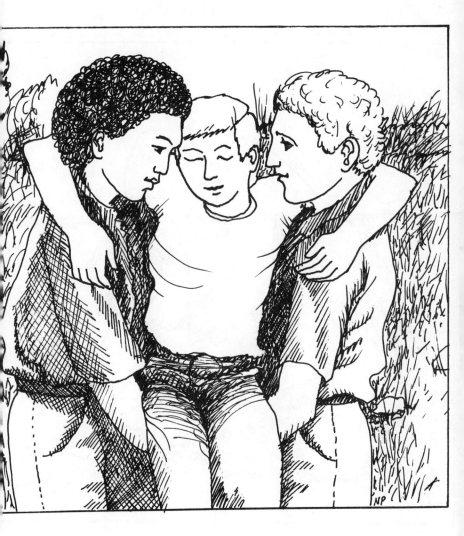

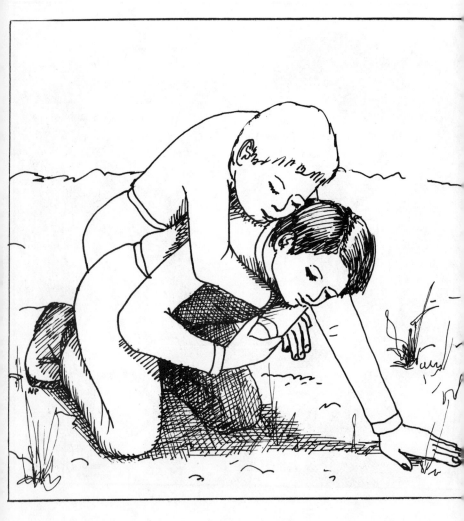

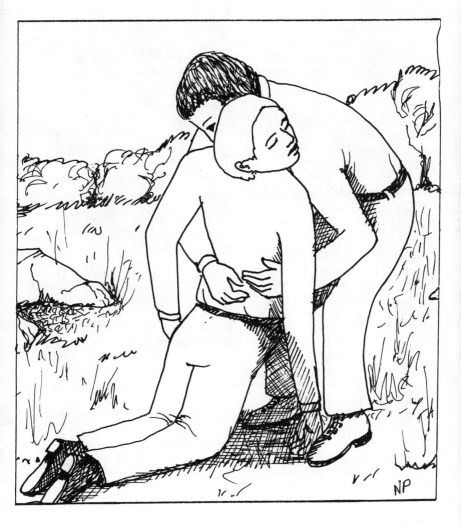

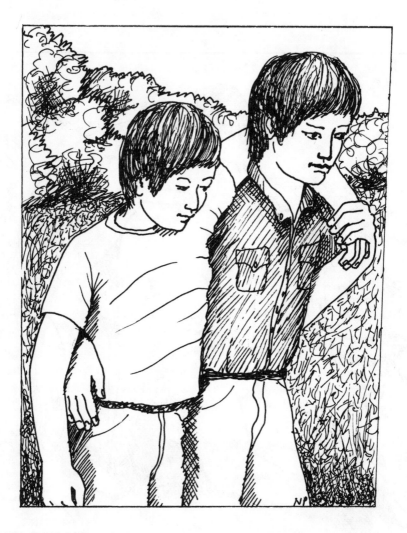

First, don't get excited; do whatever first aid treatment is required before you try to move a victim. This means splinting any fractures, stopping any bleeding and treating for shock. The decision to move anyone with a fracture or suspected fracture of the neck or spine must be seriously considered and done only in the most extreme emergency.

BROKEN NECK

A stretcher is no good for moving anyone with a broken neck or back. Stretchers are far too flexible. You will need to build a combination splint and stretcher from 2 x 6 or wider boards with cross braces where the feet, hips and shoulder will be and pad the boards with whatever might be at hand. If the victim is already lying on his back put the stretcher beside him. You will need people to help you so that the victim can be lifted and the stretcher put under him without twisting the head, neck or spine in any way. This is very important. If you are sloppy at this point the victim may be a coroner's case instead of a hospital emergency. If the victim is lying on his stomach, or side, very carefully roll him to a face up position on the stretcher and tie him to it securely with his head held stationary between supports.

Move a victim with a broken back in the same way as with a broken neck, except face down. If he is lying all or partially on his back already, it could be best to attach him to a splint before turning him on his stomach.

As a last resort, a blanket stretcher may be used as shown.

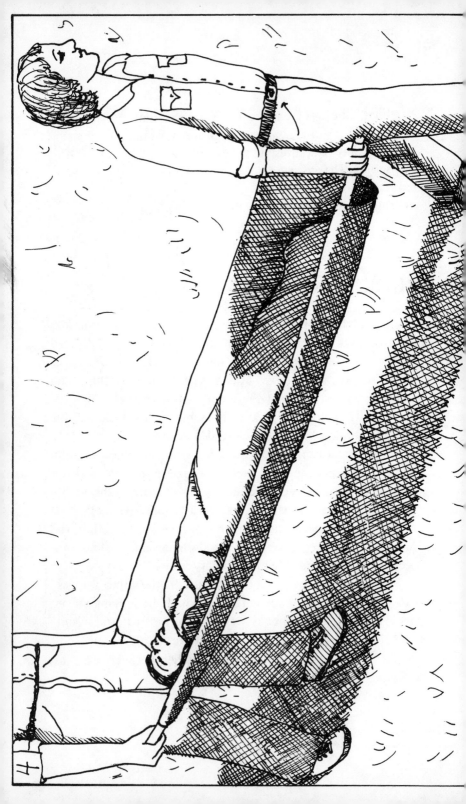

If you do not have enough help or the right things to use, it may be better to not move anyone with a broken neck or back.

In other types of injuries a stretcher is an ideal way of moving someone.

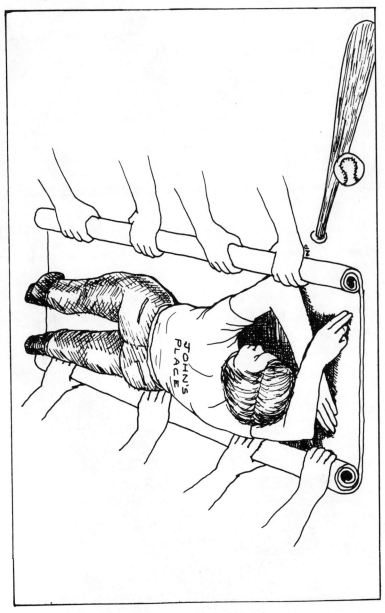

Obviously a standard, ordinary everyday stretcher, which nobody ever has when it is needed, is the best. In some places, though, it might take a week to find one.

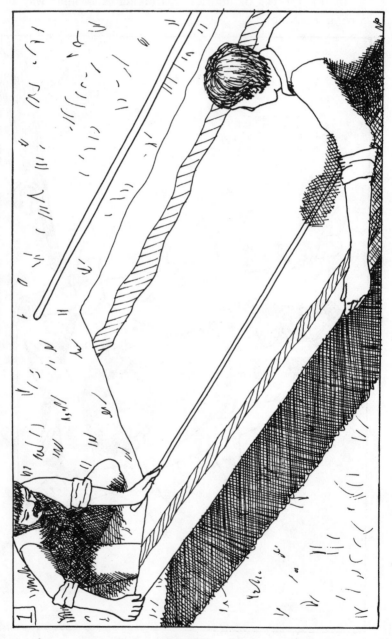

A suitable stretcher may be made from a blanket, tarp or chicken wire and a couple of strong poles, as shown below.

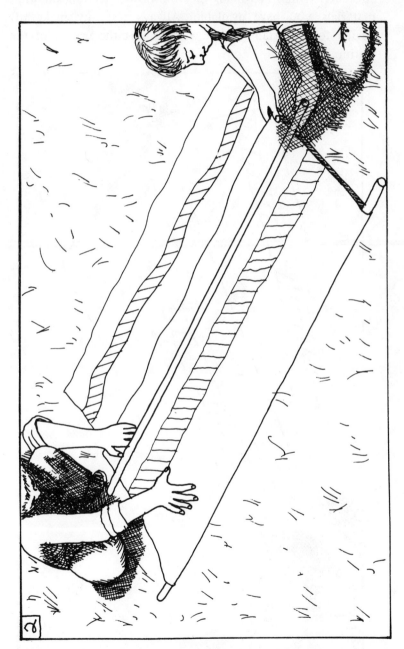

A door, a ladder, a gate or a plank may also be used as a stretcher. There are many possibilities depending on what materials you have available. Always test any makeshift device to be certain that it will support the weight of the victim.

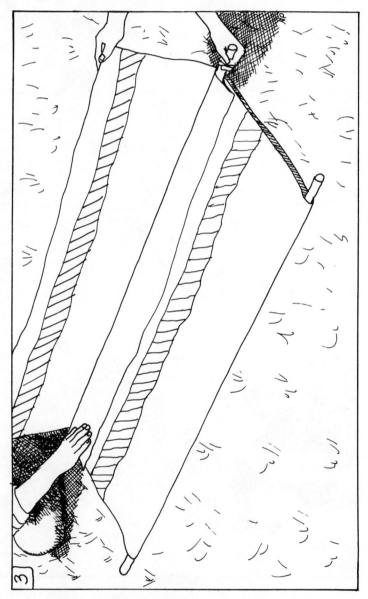

FOREIGN OBJECT IN EYE

Working around trees with chain saws or axes, handling hay or underbrush, or any number of miscellaneous homestead activities, there is a pretty fair chance of getting something in your eye. Nature has provided us with a good flushing system of tears and involuntary blinking that will dislodge most small particles from under the eyelids, but now and then a little outside help is called for. The first important rule is: Don't rub the eye. You could scratch the surface of the eyeball or damage the cornea.

If the foreign object is lodged under the lower lid, have the person look upward. Then, firmly and gently, pull the lower lid downward until the object can be seen. Be sure your hands are clean. With the tip of the corner of a clean handkerchief, cloth or shirt-tail, the object can be carefully touched and swept away. If the cloth is slightly damp, it will help the object stick to the cloth when it touches.

If the object is under the upper lid, the person should look downward while the upper lid is carefully lifted up and out. The edge of a match stick or the side of a pencil can be placed over the lid so it can be rolled upward to reveal the offending matter. The moist corner of the handkerchief should do the trick.

If the object adheres to the cornea of the eye (the lens), it's a good idea to have the patient blink until it moves so that no damage is done to that very sensitive and delicate area.

In case the object seems to be imbedded into the surface of the eyeball, it is best not to try to remove it yourself, assuming you can get to a doctor fairly soon. Cover the eye lightly with a moist cotton wad or clean cloth and secure it with a bandage or bandana.

If the eyeball has been scratched, it may feel as though the object is still there. Rinse the eye with water or boric acid, using moist cotton and a loose bandage until the irritation lessens to a tolerable state.

139

GUNSHOT WOUNDS

Despite the fact that many modern-day homesteaders are opposed to having firearms around, the gunshot wound still remains a possibility. Some of the most peace-loving anti-gun people have finally resorted to keeping a gun on hand to protect their poultry and livestock from marauding varmints. And, of course, there are others who have guns. In the wilderness there are many instances of trigger-happy deer hunters who have, in their eagerness, shot cows, autos, scarecrows, dogs and folks.

Those people who are inexperienced with firearms may not have learned that a gun should be kept unloaded when not being fired, and should never be pointed at anyone, even when it is believed to be unloaded. Accidents do happen, and it's not a bad idea to know what steps to take with bullet wounds.

First of all, with any gunshot wound, you should assume that the wound is contaminated and that infection might occur. Clean the wound as thoroughly as possible, using a mild disinfectant so as not to burn the tissue or inhibit coagulation.

Unless the bullet is clearly visible at the surface of the flesh, and easily removed, it should be left for a surgeon to remove as quickly as you can get to him. Digging deeply into the victim's flesh could cause severe and unnecessary pain and bleeding, as well as increase the chances of infection.

Stop the bleeding, as with any other type of wound, and do your best to alleviate any kind of breathing difficulties. Unless the wound has damaged the breathing apparatus, it's usually a good idea to elevate the feet a few inches. In the event that a lung or windpipe has been punctured, do your best to plug the escaping air with wadding and have the patient lie on the side which has been wounded.

In most cases, gunshot wounds are going to require some degree of surgery, in which case the patient should be given no food or liquids for several hours prior to the operation.

Remember, too, that the bullet might have struck and fractured a bone. Try to determine if such is the case, and be careful in moving the victim not to compound the problem. If you think a bone has been damaged, use splints, just in case, and treat the patient for broken bones as described elsewhere in this book. Although it may seem unlikely, even gunshot wounds have been known to cause bone fractures, especially at close range.

In cases of short-range gunshot injuries, there is a pretty good likelihood of painful powder burns on the flesh in addition to the bullet wound. Even blanks can inflict severe powder burns. Clean the burn as well as you can to relieve the pain and to reduce the possibility of infection.

CONCLUSION

Whatever injuries or disorders may be suffered, let's try to remember that the human body is equipped with a rather miraculous ability to heal itself. Fear and panic are inclined to interfere with the natural healing processes. Remember, there are direct electro-chemical connections between the thinking mind and the cells, tissues, nerves and organs of the body. It is a known fact that the autonomic nervous system carries thought messages to all parts of the body. These messages have a profound effect upon the body's ability to muster the necessary powers of natural healing. Let the injured person be calmed and reassured that his body knows what to do. Help him to maintain a quiet confidence in his automatic life forces and natural healing powers. A positive pro-life attitude will go a long way toward a swift recovery.

BACK, broken — 125
BEE stings — 93
BIRTH — 63
BLEEDING wounds
  — 7
BLEEDING nose
  — 17
BONES, broken
  — 113
BREACH birth — 83
BROKEN bones
  — 113
BRONCHITIS — 58
CHARLIE horse
  — 109

CHEMICAL poison-
  ing — 39
CHILDBIRTH — 63
CHILDHOOD
  accidents — 55
CHOKING — 23
COLDS — 57
COLLARBONE,
  broken — 123
CONVULSIONS
  — 59
CRAMPS, heat — 53
EARACHE — 58
ELBOW, broken
  — 119

ELECTRICAL
shock — 101
EXTERNAL heart
massage — 29
EYE, foreign object
in — 139
FINGER, broken
— 122
FIRST aid kit — 5
FOOD poisoning
— 37
FOOT, broken
— 116
FOREIGN bodies
in eye — 62
FROSTBITE — 54
GUNSHOT wound
— 140
HAND, broken
— 121
HEAD, concussion
— 127
HEAD injuries — 59

HEART massage
— 29
KNEE cap, broken
— 117
MOUTH-to-mouth
rescuscitation — 19
MUSHROOM poison-
ing — 33
NECK, broken
— 125, 133
NOSE bleeds — 17
PELVIS, broken
— 124
POISON oak, ivy,
sumac — 104
POISON snake
bites — 87
POISONING:
acid —·45
aspirin — 49
alkalies — 46
carbolic acid — 45
chemical — 39

creosole — 45
food — 37
strychnine — 47
PNEUMONIA — 58
PRESSURE points
  — 8
PULSE — 104
RESCUSCITATION
  — 19
RIBS, broken — 123
SALMONELLA
  poisoning — 39
SCORPIONS — 96
SHOCK — 99
SHOCK, electrical
  — 101
SNAKEBITE — 85
SPIDERS — 95

SPRAINS — 107
STRAINS — 107
SUNBURN — 51
SUNSTROKE — 52
THIGH, broken
  — 118
TICKS — 97
TOES, broken — 116
TOURNIQUET — 13
TRANSPORTATION
  — 127
WOUNDS, bleeding
  — 7
WOUNDS, gunshot
  — 140
WOUNDS, puncture
  — 16
WRIST, broken
  — 121

OLIVER PRESS BOOKS

JOSEPH ROSENBLOOM
Kits and Plans
Finder's Guide No. 1

Where to purchase plans and kits for practically anything you can think of. From mini-bikes to harpsichords, this guide tells who offers what and what it costs. *288 pages*

ISBN 0-914400-00-2   Price $3.95 paper

JOSEPH ROSENBLOOM
Craft Supplies Supermarket
Finder's Guide No. 2

An illustrated and indexed directory of craft supplies. Thousands of products including materials, kits, tools from over 450 companies are analyzed from their catalogs. *Index, illustrations, 224 pages*

ISBN 0-914400-01-0   Price $3.95 paper

ANNE HECK
The Complete Kitchen
Finder's Guide No. 3

A comprehensive guide to hard-to-find utensils. This book describes the companies supplying such utensils as well as offering information on their catalogs. *Illustrated, 96 pages*

ISBN 0-914400-02-9   Price $2.95 paper

GARY WADE
Homegrown Energy
Power for the Home and Homestead
Finder's Guide No. 4

A complete directory to the thousands of available products involved in the production of home grown power. Water wheels, solar cells, windmills and other exotic equipment are covered and indexed in depth. *Illustrated, 96 pages*

ISBN 0-914400-03-7   Price $2.95 paper

ARMAND BITEAUX
The New Consciousness
Finder's Guide No. 5

A guide to spiritual groups: name; address, international, national, local; statement of philosophy; biographies of leaders; bibliography of publications of the group. *Index, 176 pages*

ISBN 0-914400-04-5   Price $3.95 paper

ROLAND ROBERTSON
Spices, Condiments, Teas, Coffees, and Other Delicacies
Finder's Guide No. 6

This illustrated and indexed directory answers difficult questions involved with finding and purchasing unusual ingredients, beverages and foods which are difficult to obtain locally. *Index, illustrated, 208 pages*

ISBN 0-914400-05-3   Price $3.95 paper

FRED DAVIS
Country Tools
Essential Hardware and Livery
Finder's Guide No. 7

Locates sources for otherwise difficult-to-find tools essential to country living. This indispensible guide to the country resident working his land covers everything from bell scrapers to goat harnesses to spoke shavers. *Illustrated, 160 pages*

ISBN 0-914400-06-1   Price $3.95 paper

PAT FALGE and ARNOLD LEGGETT
The Complete Garden
Finder's Guide No. 8

The catalogs of over 400 garden tool and seed companies which sell
by mail order organized into a comprehensive guide. From carrots to
kohlrabi, from tomato stakes to rabbit repellent, it tells who sells what
and how to get it. *Illustrated, 256 pages*
ISBN 0-914400-11-8   Price $3.95 paper

DERWOOD McCRAKEN
Mother Nature's Recipe Book
Mother Nature Series No. 1

Includes some 70 commonly found wild plants with detailed draw-
ings of each plant and recipes for preparing a main course from each.
Plant identification is emphasized as are tested, nutritional meals which
can contribute to the average household's fight against rising food costs.
Illustrated, 160 pages
ISBN 0-914400-07-X   Price $3.95 paper

DEZIRINA GOUZIL
Mother Nature's Herbs and Teas
Mother Nature Series No. 2

A guide to approximately 112 easily found herbs and other plants
that are used in the preparation of seasonings and beverages. This introduction for the layman includes detailed illustrations of each plant and
a description of its habitat. *Illustrated, 256 pages*
ISBN 0-914400-08 8   Price $3.95 paper

WILL BEARFOOT
Mother Nature's Dyes and Fibers
Mother Nature Series No. 3

A book of plants and trees utilized in the preparation of dyes and weaving materials by North American Indians. The author has drawn his research from interviews with Indians still using the original methods. Step-by-step procedures are outlined and accompanied by detailed illustrations of the plants and trees used. *Illustrated, 160 pages*
ISBN 0-914400-10-X   Price $3.95 paper

DR. JUDY WILSON
Mother Nature's Homestead First Aid
Mother Nature Series No. 4

This book is a rural emergency first aid tool, emphasizing self-help procedures for everything from sprains to major injuries. It is indispensible for those who live in remote areas with little access to professional medical help. Special attention is given to the preparation of the sick or injured for transportation to medical facilities. *Illustrated, 160 pages*
ISBN 0-914400-09-6   Price $3.95 paper

MICHAEL BARLEYCORN
Moonshiner's Manual

A do-it-yourself detailed guide to making your own whiskey. Laws of the fifty states and the Federal government are included along with chapters on history, recipes, safety and chemistry—all written in an easy to understand, delightfully entertaining manner. *Illustrated, 160 pages*
ISBN 0-914400-12-6   Price $3.95 paper